The Island

The Island
Nurse

MARY J. MACLEOD

MAINSTREAM
PUBLISHING
EDINBURGH AND LONDON

First published in Great Britain in 2012 by
MAINSTREAM PUBLISHING COMPANY
(EDINBURGH) LTD
7 Albany Street
Edinburgh EH1 3UG

ISBN 9781845967901

This book is a work of non-fiction based on the life, experiences and recollections of the author. In some cases, names of people, places, dates, sequences or the details of events have been changed to protect the privacy of others. The author has stated to the publisher that, except in such cases, not affecting the substantial accuracy of the work, the contents of the book are true.

A catalogue record for this book is available
from the British Library

Printed in Great Britain by Clays Ltd, St Ives plc

5 7 9 10 8 6

This book is dedicated to the memory of
Lilly Mae,
18 October 2008

Acknowledgements

I would like to thank my husband, children and friends for their interest and help (particularly my 'techno-wizard'), and the people of the island for just being themselves.

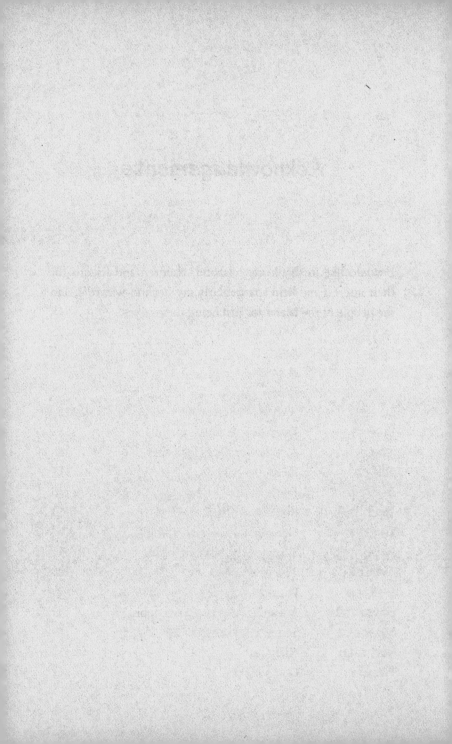

Contents

PROLOGUE

Nostalgia

Yesterday, I dozed in the garden and dreamed of the remote Hebridean island of Papavray. Quite why would be hard to say, as it is many years since I lived there, and now I am sitting in the warmth of a Cornish summer. The wild, exposed islands of the north are a far cry from Cornwall's mild and gentle weather.

So why do I feel homesick when I listen to the 'Hebrides Overture'? Why after so long do I smell peat smoke as it rises in blue snakes from the white chimneys of tiny croft houses? And feel the soft, damp air on my face and see again purple mountains, tumultuous seas and small, nameless islands in the bays?

Perhaps it's the birdsong? The skylarks are singing now. When they arrived on Papavray, it was a sign that spring was here and the brief but beautiful summer was not far behind.

I have a sudden feeling of nostalgia and instead of the colours of the garden I see the outline of the islands, behind which the sun sets in a blaze of gold, turning the rocks to pinks and reds, and the sea to shimmering amber, before sinking to leave the quiet scene to the long northern twilight. I remember the sights, sounds and smells of Papavray so well that it might have been only yesterday that I lived there, instead of all those years ago.

We had long cherished a dream of something better than our frenetic lifestyle in the south of England: something gentler, uncluttered. Perhaps returning to the land of George's forefathers?

For years it was just a dream, but this was a dream that came true!

ONE

On Papavray

It was a dreary December afternoon in 1970 as I struggled up the slippery path to the croft house on the hill above. My blue uniform and the silly hat that I had anchored with a very non-uniform scarf were no protection against the rain that was being hurled in from the sea by the blustery wind. I was cold and wet, but I knew that a cheery welcome and a warm fire awaited me, and after I had attended to my elderly patient her sister would bustle about to give me a 'wee cuppie'.

I paused on the steep slope to get my breath, pretending, as I always did, that I was just admiring the view. And what a view! Even in this weather, the island was beautiful in its wild, rugged way.

Papavray is a remote Hebridean island about 20 miles long. Numerous lochs take great bites out of the coastline so that you are never out of sight of the sea. Today, that sea was turbulent with white-topped waves crashing noisily on the rocks, sending spumes of spray far into the air. The mountains on the neighbouring islands were softly clothed in floating tendrils of mist.

Above the noise of the wind, I could hear the excited voices of young children. Wiping the rain from my eyelashes, I glanced at my watch. The little school on a nearby promontory was breaking up for Christmas and, as arranged, my youngest son, Andrew, would soon be meeting me at my patient's house. A year ago, when we moved here, he had joined the 14 other pupils of the island's only primary school and had already begun to acquire the sibilance and lilt of the gentle island tongue. He was making friends but had one big disadvantage – he did not 'have the Gaelic'. One does not speak Gaelic – one 'has the Gaelic'. Or not, in our case! It was 1970, but the more remote Scottish islands still retained this as their first language. Most of my older patients spoke a rather quaint form of English as their second language, while some spoke only their native tongue.

I climbed on up to the croft house above and knocked on the door. Of course I had been observed from the moment my car drew up on the narrow track far below, but I still found it difficult to just walk into people's houses in the manner of the locals. Calling a greeting, I stepped inside and removed my sodden coat, hat and gloves. I even took my shoes off, as they both contained a small lake of rainwater. I had not yet completed a year as the district nurse on Papavray, and I still had some notion of looking 'smart' when on my rounds. Later, I would learn that welly boots were better than shoes and that umbrellas were useless in the wind but good as walking sticks on slippery slopes and for fending off territorially minded dogs.

'Come away in, Nurse, and warm yourself by the fire. Indeed, it's terrible weather we're having the day.' This was Mary-Ann's delightful greeting as I dripped my way inside.

Minnie, my dear old patient, was in the downstairs bedroom. 'Ach, Nurse. You'll be gie wet. And so busy you are, and me here needin a bath.' I usually got her up in the mornings to sit by the fire, but today was bed-bath day.

'I'm sorry to be so late, Minnie.'

'Ach, I'm no mindin. I have my wireless.'

Minnie was almost completely paralysed as the result of a stroke some years previously, but she never complained. Over time, we became much more than nurse and patient, and when she died I felt that I had lost a friend. On this December day, we laughed and chatted as I worked, and after a while I heard Andrew's arrival. The timid knock and shy 'Hello' were followed by much motherly tutting over his wet things. Mary-Ann loved children and, like so many island women, was never happier than when fussing over them with cocoa and clootie dumpling, so Andrew was only too happy to accompany me on my rounds when necessary. The patients and their relatives plied him with all manner of goodies. I believe they thought that I didn't feed him very well. I was English, and the islanders had little regard for 'fancy English food'. Good old-fashioned stodge was what had kept them full for generations.

Nicholas, my 12 year old, a much sturdier boy, had been about to start at the senior school a year ago, just as we left the bustle of life in the south for the peace and tranquillity of Papavray. So, instead, he now attended the grammar school that served several islands and the area of mainland where it was situated. Sixty miles by road and as many more by ferry meant that he and two others from our remote village had to stay in the school hostel or in 'digs' from Monday to Friday of each week. At first he hated this but settled eventually, never becoming a good scholar but using his personality to get him by. He was very popular with old and young alike, and as a tall lad with a cheerful grin he did not want for girlfriends – even at the tender age of 12! Nicholas and Andrew were five years apart but were great friends: every weekend would see them fishing or boating or roaming far and wide. They helped the shepherds with the shearing, watched calves being born or just sat at various firesides listening to crofters' tales. It was a very different childhood from that which they would have known in the south. Our two older children were not with us on the island, having left home before we moved. Elizabeth was in college in London while John had left another college after a term, having decided that the academic life was not for him. He had a job of sorts and lived with a group of friends in the capital.

My husband, George, had been completing an overseas contract, but when he finally came to live in Dhubaig, our village, he became a sort of Jack-of-all-things-electrical for the island. We were afforded much amusement by the crofters' plaintive requests for George to breathe new life into various dying devices. Electricity had only come to the islands in 1950 and many remote glens still had none, so most of the crofters' electrical possessions had been purchased in the first excitement, and 20 years later they still expected them all to work perfectly. How often were we told 'This was a good, good kettle'? Interestingly, many of the croft houses had electric irons, kettles and so on but still no indoor toilet. I knew of two that had no toilet at all! During one summer, I gained intimate knowledge of this deficiency as a result of too many cups of tea.

As Andrew and I stood in the little hall, pulling on our still-wet coats, we could see that the rain had stopped. A huge silver moon was on the horizon, casting its own eerie glow to join the fading light of the gloomy winter day. There was a freshness in the air that spoke of calmer, drier weather to come.

'It's going to be fine for Dad coming,' Andrew said, echoing my thoughts.

George was coming home for Christmas and would be with us some time the next day – weather permitting, of course. He had flown in from South Africa and was driving up from Heathrow in time for our second Christmas on Papavray and our first in our house: we had lived in a caravan while the rebuilding took place.

'And Nick and Elizabeth and John,' continued Andrew excitedly, as we hurried to the car. The family invasion this year would include Elizabeth's latest boyfriend, Jeff . . . or was it Jim? Or Paul?

'And Nurse Robertson is coming to do your work over Christmas, isn't she?' Andrew was jumping down the hill in leaps and bounds. 'And you won't be called out or anything, will you?' he added anxiously.

I shook my head. No night calls for five days. What bliss!

We drove the eight or nine miles over the hills to the wilder side of the island, to our home in its acre or so of land facing the sea and the distant mountains. The sky had cleared and the winding road was bright in the moonlight, while the dark waters of small lochs sparkled among the reeds. Twinkling lights showed from the other islands and the moon was painting a silver path across the sea.

Later that evening, when both boys had gone to bed, I sat alone by a huge peat fire. I was sleepy but determined to catch up on my photo albums. I have kept a chronological record of our lives before and since our arrival on Papavray, but I am not good at putting the results into albums. In fact, I had not inserted any at all since our first sight of Papavray. There had been several packets of photos on the sideboard for some time now, and I had to get down to the task before the family arrived. They definitely did not share my enthusiasm for photos!

I sorted them into order and began to arrange them onto the pages of an album, but inevitably I began to study them, remembering the incidents and the people that they portrayed. It's like spreading newspaper over the carpet before decorating: one always crawls around reading long-outdated news. So it was with the photos.

There was the beach, the caravan and Alistair's boat. And the sunshine! What a contrast in the weather at that time, two summers ago, from the bitter cold of the night outside as I sat so cosily by my fire. Each photo evoked memories and the amazement that we had felt as events had worked steadily towards our present life.

TWO

Meeting Alistair

For a long time, we had been disillusioned with the way of life in the south of England where we lived, and George's work was pressurised and unrewarding. We had begun to cherish a dream of something better, gentler, a different environment altogether. Scotland, where George's father was from, came to the forefront of our minds. For years it was just a dream, but then, quite suddenly and unexpectedly, it came true. And it all began the very first time that we set foot on this Hebridean island.

It had been in the July of 1969 when we came to Papavray on holiday with Nicholas, Andrew and Duchess the retriever. We had parked our caravan on the grass beside a little beach with the sea shushing and lapping at the pebbles nearby.

George was a Glaswegian. His father had left Papavray to find work while still a young man and, like so many, had gone to Glasgow, where he lived, worked and died without ever returning to the place of his birth. Somehow, George had never had the urge to visit the isle of his antecedents. Until now!

Elizabeth and John had already started college by then and thought we were mad to travel so far just to 'sit on an island', as they put it. Nick and Andy had very different ideas. We had only arrived the night before but they were already pronouncing this as 'the best place in the world'.

So here we were on this quiet little beach enjoying the clear northern air. There was quite a large house in a garden nearby and two cottages appeared to be growing out of the rocks of a promontory across the bay. Apart from these buildings, we were alone, looking across the sea loch to a couple of islets and away to distant mountains. The setting sun was sending slanting bronze light across the water, burnishing the tops of the waves as they broke against the far shores. I could smell the peat smoke that was rising in blue snakes from the white chimneys of the two cottages.

We had wondered, with our southern conditioning, if we would be allowed to park on the beach, but as we were self-sufficient for two days, carrying twenty gallons of water and had the all-important loo, we were cautiously hopeful. However, the flimsy and all-too-obvious loo tent fell victim to the wind after only one day's use.

We had become aware, during the night, of an odd slapping noise on the side of the caravan in the blustery wind. On peering out of the window, I was just in time to see the loo tent heave itself upward, break its guy ropes and leap into the air. Like a kite in the hands of an amateur, it touched down twice before disappearing skywards. We thought of attempting a rescue but on opening the door to the gale quickly decided otherwise.

When morning came, we awoke to chuckles and some rather rude remarks from the boys, who were looking out of the window. The chemical toilet was sitting in lonely splendour on the beach like some unsophisticated throne of a minor potentate, while some of the toilet roll was attempting to wrap itself around it as though trying to clothe its nakedness. The rest of it was in small pieces that were fluttering damply over the pebbles and out to sea like so many demented seagulls. Later, on a boating trip to the islets, we found the tent draped like a pall over a large rock. It was beyond repair. Luckily, we were invited to put the loo in a nearby shed!

On a leisurely walk later that day, I stood and watched a large yacht sailing up the sea loch. Little did I know then how much this boat, or rather its occupant, would change our lives.

It was a rather luxurious boat, and I watched as it glided into the bay. It anchored and, after some delay, a dinghy was lowered, packages appeared and were stowed and then a none-too-nimble figure got in and the craft began chugging towards the shore. He made landfall at a little jetty and started to unpack the dinghy. George and the boys joined me and we ran along the path to offer assistance. Or were we just being nosy? In any case, our offer was accepted with alacrity.

The boat owner lived in the house with the garden, and it proved to be up about 30 steps. We puffed and groaned our way up with boxes and packages to find ourselves in a beautiful garden. Real gardens are rare in the islands, as the harsh weather, poor soil, ravages of deer, rabbits, cows, foxes and every other living thing makes the growing of anything other than potatoes almost impossible. But this was a gardener's garden. We collapsed onto a stone bench, hot and breathless. We all introduced ourselves.

Alistair Macphee had the typical short, stocky shape of the Highland hill-dweller, his appearance belying a precise English accent. Clad in a navy-blue jersey and seaman's cap and sporting a large moustache, his teeth were firmly clamped round an empty pipe.

'Come in, come in! We all need a dram after that,' he announced, without removing the pipe. Having spent several days alone on his boat, Alistair was ready to chat, so, packages forgotten, we settled down to hear his life story.

He had been born on the island during the First World War and lived among the local children until the age of eight, when his father decided to leave Papavray to start a business in the south of England. Alistair grew up there, and when he reached adulthood he took over his father's business and became quite wealthy. However, he never lost touch with Papavray, and when he was nearing 50 he decided to retire to his native island and put managers in to run the business.

So he built this lovely home and travelled to London occasionally to keep an eye on the business but always returned with a sense of relief. He said that Papavray was civilised and London was barbaric. Alice, his wife, whom we met later, was the gardener.

That day, as we sat in this lovely house and gazed across the sunlit bay to the hills and mountains beyond, our dream was still just that . . . a dream. Of living somewhere like this, of becoming a part of a slower way of life, of waking to the sound of the wind or the birds instead of listening to ten-ton trucks rumbling past.

Of course, there were enormous difficulties. Work, somewhere to live, education for the boys. But now we were talking to Alistair. And that made all the difference. He entered into the spirit of our aspirations with enthusiasm.

As far as work was concerned, we knew that you could tend sheep, fish, grow potatoes and so on, but these were not options for us. Whilst we were prepared to do without luxuries, we did not want poverty. George was used to designing and installing computerised control gear for large industrial concerns all over the globe. Had we been talking with a crofter, he would have felt that the sheep-tending or fishing was all that we should require. Someone from the south with a conventional background, on the other hand, might not understand why we wanted to relocate to the far north at all. But here was Alistair, who understood both points of view. An islander by birth and inclination, he knew well the pull of that way of life, but, being an erstwhile businessman, he also appreciated our expectations of that life: a decent standard for the boys, a comfortable home and enough for some of the finer things of life, not just a pound left over when the bills were paid.

If George was prepared to do basic electrical work, said Alistair, like house wiring and installing radar and sonar equipment on fishing boats, with a possible departure into the erection of TV aerials . . .We looked surprised at this, but it seemed that the first television signals were only just reaching the island.

He puffed ruminatively on a pipe that had several dead matches sprouting from its bowl. We were to learn that he very rarely smoked tobacco, only dead matches, so inexpert was he at lighting his pipe.

Looking doubtfully at me, he said, 'Do you do anything?'

Did I do anything? Apart from having four children, George's invalid mother to look after, a husband who was rarely at home, a dog, two cats, a caravan and a large house and garden, I also had a job as a nurse/health visitor! Did I *do* anything???

'Hmmm,' he said. 'Nursing, eh?' Nodding sagely, he continued, 'Yes, I think that between you, you could make a living. A modest one maybe but, yes, you could do it!'

We drew deep breaths. Could we? Dare we? Was this what we had been dreaming about for so long? It would mean leaving financial security, selling our house and abandoning everything we knew. But Alistair had given us hope.

With many thanks, we departed for our tiny home on the beach. George and I talked into the night but eventually decided that the first thing to do would be to see if there was any hope of finding somewhere to live. If that proved impossible then there was no point in agonising. And it could easily have proved impossible. We knew that under crofting laws the crofts were passed from one generation to the next. They were never sold because the land belonged to the laird even though the crofters owned the houses and outbuildings. With the diminishing population, however, many crofters had inherited more than one croft and, while they jealously guarded the land, they often had no use for the extra house. So an acre or so around the house would be fenced off and sold as a 'feu' – the name for almost anything that wasn't a croft. But so feudal was the system that not only had the laird to approve the sale but he and his minions had the power to accept or reject the potential buyer. Meetings were held where the character, lifestyle, probable usefulness and even the religious background of these individuals was probed. So even if we decided to become middle-aged dropouts (Elizabeth's words) we'd be very lucky to find anyone willing to sell us a piece of land and even luckier to be accepted into the community.

We slept poorly that night, but the next day an extraordinary thing happened which made us think that fate was taking a hand.

THREE

A 'small acre'

We had driven along the little coastal lane from the beach to find a phone box. Beth had been taking exams at college and we wanted to find out how she had fared. We reached Dhubaig (although we did not know the name of the scattered little township at that time) without seeing any sign of a phone, so we looked around for someone to ask.

Standing beside the road was a crofter, very weatherbeaten, and his wife who was wearing a bright apron. They were feeding some chickens and regarding us with frank curiosity. This part of Papavray was so remote and the road so primitive that the appearance of any strangers aroused immediate interest. We asked about the phone and, with much gesturing, they pointed to what looked like a tin hut but which, they assured us, was the post office. We chatted and with some self-conscious hesitancy we expressed our half-formed hopes that we might be able to live here one day. An odd glance passed between the crofter and his wife.

Taking courage, George blurted out, 'Do you know if anyone has a house or land for sale?'

'Yes, I have!'

For just a second, the world stood still. I was sure of it! I was suddenly acutely aware of the birdsong and the smell of the damp earth. Was this a coincidence or a minor miracle? Or fate? I stole a glance at George. He was staring at the blue-eyed, wind-reddened face of the crofter.

'Well, I . . . um . . .' George was lost for words.

Mr Crofter was looking at his boots and shuffling his feet. I felt then, and continued to feel, that, on Papavray, negotiations of any sort were conducted through a fog of half-understood cultural differences.

'Well, y'see, old Morag passed over some time back and she'd no bairns to her and no relatives foreby. No. She left the croft to go back and I got it from the factor.'

Trying to unravel this information was as bad as untangling Andrew's fishing lines, but I was impatient to see the house, so I didn't ask for an explanation.

'It's not a croft, y'understand, but I can let you have the house and a wee bit land on a feu.'

Although Alistair had attempted our education on the subject of 'feus', I was still rather hazy about the difference between a feu and a croft. Indeed, everyone called our property a croft anyway.

'Come away in and have a cuppie,' piped Mrs Crofter. No introductions had been made on their side, so we had no idea of their names.

The last thing I wanted to do was to chat over a cup of tea. I wanted to see the house and this 'feu' thing, but courtesy demanded that we accompany them into their home.

A scaldingly hot cup of tea was served in chipped but once-best teacups with saucers. When we got to know these people better and were accepted into the community, we were given older cups with more chips and no saucers. The conversation ranged over the usual themes of the weather, the tides, the sheep – everything except the house. It was as though once the offer had been made, as it were, the subject was closed for the time being. Looking back, I can now see that they had probably already said too much, as the laird had not been approached for his permission to divide up this croft that our crofter had somehow wangled into his possession.

We eventually persuaded Archie and Mary, as they turned out to be called, to show us the house. They led us through a small gate and across a long narrow croft of about three acres. At the opposite end was a miserable, dilapidated building with a rusty corrugated-iron roof, rotting door and filthy windows. Approached by no path or road of any kind, it stood among the tussocky grass and rugged boulders, staring out across the valley to the distant mountains.

The village of Dhubaig was not like most others that we had seen, which had been arranged along the glen roads; this one had no shape or logic to the distribution of the little white blobs that were the houses. It was as if God had tossed a handful of white pebbles into the glen that dipped away below us. The heather-clad hills rose on three sides and the sea formed the fourth. A stream tumbled down the hill behind the house and wandered away over the croft to water thirsty animals on its way to the shore, where it chattered fussily over the pebbles and into the waiting sea. Standing sentinel on a headland across the bay were the ruins of a castle.

'Will we go into the house, then?'

At last!

Archie pushed open the drooping door: no key, of course. No handle either. In we went to a tiny hall with doors on either side and a rough, ladder-like stair rising in front of us. We entered the room on the right. Concrete floor, wood-lined walls, a fireplace and ample signs of its present use as a store for animal feed. Several musty-smelling sacks of knobbly, unidentifiable objects were stacked against one wall. The room on the left was a great deal worse!

'This is the room,' announced Mary. So far as I could see, they were both rooms of a sort. I must have looked puzzled.

'The other one is the kitchen. This one's "the room".' Mary considered this to be sufficient explanation.

Later, I learnt that the early crofts had only two rooms: the kitchen and the bedroom. The later ones were built with a rudimentary bedroom upstairs, so the second downstairs room became something of an embarrassment, as no one knew what to use it for or what to call it. So it was 'the room that wasn't a kitchen', later contracted to simply 'the room'.

I ascended the ladder/stairs to the open space above. A boarded floor and a skylight and that was it! No bathroom, no toilet and downstairs no kitchen as we know it. Just the two rooms, such as they were. No electricity, no drainage (there was nothing to drain anyway) and one tap. And that was outside. Some house!

But . . . as I looked out of the skylight, a skein of geese flew past and across the glen a young girl started to play the bagpipes, standing at the end of her cottage on the hill. The sky was clearing in places and shafts of silver-yellow sunlight streamed over the far mountains, picking out the jagged peaks against a blue/black, inky sky. As I watched, two people greeted each other on the road down in the valley, stopping to talk, and had I been able to understand the Gaelic I could have heard every word: the village was so quiet.

George was prowling about outside, looking at the byre, the stream and the land around the house.

A 'small acre'

'And how much land would we get with the house?' he asked.

'Well, I'm needing the land for the cow and the oats. Then there's the lambing . . .' Archie was hedging. He obviously did not want to let us have much land.

'What about an acre?' queried George.

'Oh. No, no. Indeed no. Not as much as an acre! I couldna spare an acre.'

'Oh, well then, I don't know . . .' George left the sentence in mid-air. I was scared for a moment, thinking that he really would decide against the whole thing if he couldn't get his acre. Did he know how much I wanted this? Did he feel the same?

'Ach, well . . .' Archie kicked a stone.

Mary put a stop to this merry-go-round by saying firmly, 'Well, you could have a small acre.'

'What's going on, Mum? Dad?'

Nick and Andy had returned from discovering the stream and its possibilities. The boys now stood side by side, viewing the house with some horror.

'The island is great and so is the village, but we can't live in that!' announced Nick.

But Andy was beginning to develop opinions of his own. He addressed Nick.

'They'll get it fixed.' He turned, 'Won't you, Mum?'

'Of course,' I assured them. 'Would you like to live here?'

'Oh yes!' they replied in unison. Then a worried frown creased Nick's brow. 'What about school?'

Ah! In the south of England in 1969, 11 year olds were sent where the education authority decreed: there was no choice. This was one of the things about which we were unhappy.

'Alistair told us that the senior school is on the mainland. Pupils living a long way off have to stay in the school hostel during the week. Would you mind that?'

'Mmm . . . it might be fun . . . but . . .'

He sounded doubtful, as well he might. It would be a big change at an impressionable age, but we were convinced that it would be a better option than the tough school that he was due to attend.

'We'll talk about it all, I promise,' I said. 'Don't worry about it.'

They didn't. They rushed off to explore the shore and watch a boat coming into the bay. The bay that gave the village its name: Dhubaig. 'Dhu' meant 'black', referring to the rocks, and 'aig' was Gaelic for 'bay'.

I wandered back to the house (in its 'small acre'), leaving Archie and George to talk about money – the part of the purchase of any property that I always found embarrassing, despite having moved many times and lived in several different countries.

Under the stairs and opening into the kitchen was a box-bed that I had not noticed in my hasty glance round the room. It was the first I had seen and appeared to be a kind of wide shelf about two feet from the floor, in a sort of cupboard. There were no doors on this, but a tattered curtain hung in front of it. Rotting bedding was still in evidence and the walls were covered in a paper depicting exotic flowers such as old Morag would never have seen. I stood beside that bed and was aware of a cold, rather strange feeling: rather like opening the door from a warm room into an unheated porch. There was a very odd atmosphere there. Even when we had rebuilt and heated the house, the cold spot persisted.

Mary had followed me and began to chatter. 'Of course, at the meeting the laird will want to know if you are going to stay here. Are you sure you don't just want it for holidays?'

I assured her that we intended to move here permanently.

'And what will your man do for work?'

I explained what 'my man' would do and added that if there was anything on the island for a trained nurse to do, maybe I could work too.

'There's a wee hospital on the other side.'

I was amused to hear her talk of the 'other side'. The phrase was so often used to describe the other side of death, and we had already heard the terms 'passing on' and 'passing over'. We did seem to be referring to death rather a lot, but I knew that 'the other side' referred to the opposite side of the high spine of hills that ran roughly down the middle of the island. Most places of importance – hospital, harbour, garage and so on – were on the other side of this steep hill. Dhubaig and Coiravaig were the only two villages on our side.

A price had been agreed between Archie and George. 'If the laird and the factor agree and the meeting lets you in,' added Archie. Mary imparted the apparently exciting news that I was a trained nurse.

Finally, we remembered the phone call, collected the boys and promised to return the following day. Elizabeth had passed with flying colours.

After some essential shopping on 'the other side', we returned to our home on the beach, taking far more notice of every hill and glen, every loch and lochan, in readiness for our residence here . . . we hoped!

The all-important meeting was scheduled for the following day. We were not invited, as I suppose they wanted freedom to talk about us rather than to us. Late in the evening, an ancient car crunched to a halt on the pebbles and Archie thundered on the door.

'It's all right,' said he. 'You have been approved!'

Apparently, this was a considerable departure from normal policy, as we were the first incomers to 'our side' of the island. There had been much heart searching and some dissenting voices before a vote decided our fate and we were allowed to contaminate the indigenous population of Dhubaig.

Archie had no understanding of the procedures to be followed in property transfers. One evening, he asked for the money for the house as though we were buying a chair or a bicycle and was amazed when we told him that solicitors and deeds were involved.

We intended to finish our holiday, go home and start negotiations to buy the feu and sell our house. Our centrally heated, modern, dry, clean, convenient house that we were leaving to buy this old, near-derelict, damp, remote wreck with no facilities! Were we quite mad?

So home we went. Our solicitor, while seeming to believe that he was dealing with folk from outer space rather than from a Hebridean island, still managed everything smoothly so that a completion date was soon arranged.

And so, one damp Friday afternoon in 1969, we came to our 'small acre'.

*

But enough of this reminiscing by the fire! I put the albums away. It was late. George was arriving in the morning and Christmas was upon us, so I should be getting to bed.

FOUR

Katy

The next day dawned at about 9.30. It was only two days past the winter solstice and, being so far north, the days were very short. George would probably arrive fairly early, as he often travelled overnight catching the early ferries, so I had been up long before it got light.

I was just stoking the Rayburn when Duchess began to wag her tail and in came George. The boys came tumbling from their beds and mayhem ensued. We had a huge breakfast and George unpacked all manner of weird presents, including an enormous sledge, and the boys started hoping for snow.

That evening, we drove to the steamer to meet John, Elizabeth and her boyfriend. There was a feeling of excitement in the air as the lights of the little ship came into view. They were waving from the deck as she drew alongside the tiny pier. Oh dear! Would I get the boyfriend's name right?

Down the gangplank they came. John immediately took Andy onto his shoulders, cuffing Nick's head by way of greeting. I received a bear hug and George endured a very firm handshake. Elizabeth appeared, more restrained, accompanied by a very tall, thin, dark-haired but blue-eyed young man who was introduced as Paul. While she hugged us all, he gazed round at the office-cum-shop-cum-store room on the narrow stone pier and at the single-track lane leading away into the darkness beyond.

People and luggage were loaded into the Land Rover and everyone talked at once on the trek homeward to a celebratory dinner. The night was cold but overcast. No moon or stars tonight.

Early the next morning, I became aware of an ominous stillness. Fearfully, I opened an eye. As I thought: instead of darkness, there was an eerie white light on the ceiling. Snow! Excited shouts came from the boys' bedrooms and downstairs a rather chilly Paul was warming himself by the Rayburn.

The snow was deep and beautiful, with huge drifts. Not a human footprint sullied the surface that was luminescent in the early light, but foxes, rabbits and deer had obviously visited us in the night. The sea looked like slate, and the sky held the promise of more snow to come. The corries on the mountains were white, but many of the peaks were too sheer for the snow to pitch and looked even more stark than usual against the glowing white of their surroundings.

A hasty breakfast and everyone was off! Snowballs and sledging were the order of the day, followed, no doubt, by steaming heaps of clothes round the Rayburn. After a hectic morning, we were about to stop for some hot soup and a warm-up when a shout caught my attention. Struggling through the deep snow towards us was an agitated figure.

'Murdoch! What's the matter?'

'Nurse! Nurse . . .' Murdoch paused to get his breath. 'It's Katy again! Come quick!'

'What about the doctor?' I queried as I loped along beside him.

'He canna come. The road's blocked. Tis Loch Annan . . .'

It was always Loch Annan, or rather the steep hill beside it.

'What's wrong with Katy?'

'She canna breathe right, and she's awful pale.'

I shouted back to Nick to fetch my bag and to John to bring my small oxygen cylinder. We were already making our way up to Murdoch's croft.

As soon as I entered the dark, smoky house, I could see that Katy, Murdoch's 22-year-old daughter, was very ill. Marion, her mother, was hovering about her. Katy had leukaemia, which had been in remission for some months but had just flared up again, and as a result of this serious blood disorder she was particularly prone to infections. We had been pumping antibiotics into her for several days, but this was bad.

'Hello, Katy. Let me sit you up a bit higher. More pillows, Marion, please?'

Marion hurried away and returned with her own and Murdoch's pillows. Between us, we raised the gasping girl and I was pleased to see that her breathing eased. But her lips were blue and she was clearly exhausted.

Nick arrived with my bag and John followed with the oxygen. I was just opening the cylinder when I noticed that Murdoch had lit a cigarette. John noticed at the same moment and startled the old man by snatching it from his mouth and hurling it out into the snow. I left John to explain about the fire risk.

I told them that I was going to ring the doctor for his advice.

'You canna. His line's gone down,' said Murdoch.

This was hopeless! There were more blue/black clouds on the horizon, and I could see that snow was falling again on one of the neighbouring islands. I looked at Katy and listened to her laboured breathing. I didn't like the look of the weather or the patient, and I had to decide what to do. There was no possibility of help from the doctor, but I knew that my phone was working. As the district nurse, I had the only phone (other than the post office) in the village. I made a decision.

Telling Marion to go on giving Katy oxygen and leaving John to monitor Murdoch's smoking habits, I floundered my way home to do the only thing now open to me. I rang the RAF Helicopter Service. Helicopter help these days is almost routine, but in the far north in the early '70s, it was very new.

'The weather's closing in,' came the doubtful reply to my request.

'It's desperate! I really believe that she will die if we cannot get immediate hospital treatment.' There was some muttering at the other end of the very crackly line.

'Can you have the patient ready and at a suitable landing spot by 1300 hours?'

Mentally changing this to real time, I said 'Yes' with more confidence than I felt. Murdoch's croft was perched on a rocky outcrop with no real access apart from a boulder-strewn, steep cliff-like path. We'd have to get her down to the flatter land in the village centre. And it was already 12.15 p.m.

The stern voice resumed. 'Right. We must be away by 13.30, as the weather window will probably close at 15.00 and we have 155 miles to do to the hospital.'

This was all pretty unreal. I drew breath.

'Fine. Middle of the village – area about the size of a school playground all right?'

'Mmm . . . any trees?'

'No trees.'

'Right. On our way.'

Katy

Leaving George to round up some of the able-bodied men in the village and tell their wives to fill hot water bottles, I fished out a warm sleeping bag and some thick socks. Elizabeth added a woolly bonnet and gloves, and everyone set off to Murdoch's croft through the snow once more.

On the way, I tried to think how we were going to get Katy down across the rocks without the aid of a stretcher. The oxygen had to come too, preferably without a break in its administration. Suppose the men slipped and dropped her? Suddenly, I caught sight of the sledge. It was huge: now it might come in useful. I grabbed it and towed it with me up and over the crag to Murdoch's house. Katy seemed fractionally better. The oxygen was helping, but she was very weak and her chest rattled alarmingly.

We set about giving her a warm drink and bundling her into the socks, pullover and bonnet. By then the men had arrived with hot water bottles and ropes. (Ropes?) The sledge was just big enough to take most of Katy's tiny body in a semi-sitting position, but her thin little legs had to stick out over the end. We strapped two pillows at her back and a man got behind to hold her up. Blankets tucked tightly around her, with the hot water bottles inside, kept her reasonably warm.

Off we went! One man on each side to hold her, one to hold her feet, John carrying the oxygen and myself generally hovering. Puffing and struggling, the men still had breath for some mild ribaldry and a lot of laughter. I have always marvelled at the ability of the average Gael to find something to laugh about in the most unlikely situation. Katy was amazingly brave throughout.

Marion joined us with a small paper carrier full of Katy's 'things', muttering about going with her daughter, but there would be two pilots and a doctor as well as the patient, leaving little space for a substantial lady like Marion.

As the procession neared the snow-covered area beside the road, we became aware of the drone of the approaching helicopter. Some of the men had had the presence of mind to arrange some tattered red curtains in the shape of a cross. The pilot circled the village, obviously checking the suitability of our makeshift helipad.

With a flurry of snow, the monster landed. We waited for the engine to die, but it continued to roar. Two figures jumped out, the badge on the uniform of the first proclaiming him to be the doctor. I went forward and we conferred by shouting within an inch of each other's ear. The other figure hovered somewhat agitatedly.

'We must be away,' he said. 'That's why we have not turned the engines off. The weather is closing in and the pilot is anxious to go.'

The pilot now appeared with earmuffs and protective clothing for Katy. With oiled expertise, she was lifted from the sledge and onto the helicopter's purpose-built stretcher and an oxygen supply was set up. She was loaded aboard and the doctor jumped in beside her. During all this, she smiled and gave a weak wave.

We were told to 'stand away', the doors were closed and we cowered away from the now-familiar blast of snow as the monster lifted into the already darkening sky. I looked at my watch: 13.30 precisely! We watched as the retreating helicopter disappeared over the hill and the noise gradually faded. The silence was almost as deafening as the engines had been.

Marion was weeping pitifully. She not been able to accompany her daughter, and because of the uncertain telephone communication she felt that she might not even hear if Katy arrived safely or how she progressed. I promised to do all that I could to keep everyone informed.

There seemed to be a sense of anticlimax and people milled around for a while, chatting and shaking their heads, before gathering their possessions and trudging homeward through the gloom. At least 20 of the 42 inhabitants of Dhubaig were present that afternoon to help Katy.

We too trudged home to get out of our wet clothes, build up the Rayburn and the now-dead fire and try to warm up. John, Nick and Andy had been very impressed with the whole procedure and the size of the helicopter with its array of instruments, which they had seen through the door. Paul must have wondered what this new girlfriend of his had got him into!

Later that evening, the phone rang. It was the hospital. Katy had arrived safely, been diagnosed as having pneumonia (no surprise to anyone), and was then sedated and put on an antibiotic drip. She was said to be 'comfortable'.

I ploughed across the valley once more to tell Marion and Murdoch the good news, and as I returned the snow began to fall again. Well, that was the first of my so-called five days off!

FIVE

A nurse's nightmare

Christmas Day was wet and windy. Our usual winter weather.

I rang my relief nurse, Nurse Robertson, to tell her about Katy and to make sure that she was able to get about the island to do the routine visits. There was no reply. I rang Dr Mac, but he had not seen her. However, the Loch Annan road was open, the doctor had been told, so I said that I would come over to do the essentials and try to locate my relief nurse.

I set out early to traverse the ten miles over the top to the nurse's house. There was slush on the road and piled beside it were walls of fast-melting packed snow. We did not warrant a snowplough (I don't think there was one on the island), but some of the men had been wielding shovels under the eye of the factor.

As I walked up to the front door of the nurse's house, it was suddenly flung open and a tall man, clearly in a terrible temper, strode out. With no more than a glance, he pushed past me on the narrow path, but as he reached the gate he appeared to take in the significance of my uniform.

'You're the other one, are you? Well, she won't be staying here!'

He strode off down the road. I was completely at a loss but most alarmed. Was she inside? What was going on?

I pushed the door open. 'Angela, are you there?'

No reply.

I advanced tentatively into the hallway. A creaking sound made me look up and there, sitting on the top stair, was my relief nurse. Her face was swollen. Her hair, usually constrained in a neat bun, was loose and unkempt, and she was wearing her dressing gown. It was bitterly cold in the house but her feet were bare.

Angela was clearly hysterical. 'I'm leaving! Now! Today! He's found me and I can't stay.'

None of this made sense. 'Angela, come and sit down. I'll switch the fire on and you come and get warm in here. Then you can tell me all about it.'

Slowly, she came down the stairs and into the sitting room.

'I can't stay,' she repeated. 'You can't make me!' She didn't seem to know who I was. Her eyes were wild and unfocused, and her movements were jerky and uncoordinated. She sat by the pathetic little electric fire like someone in a dream and stared straight ahead.

'I have to ring the doctor, Angela. We were very worried about you.'

'I'm not staying,' she said again. 'He can't make me stay here.'

I called the doctor from the hall and in almost a whisper I tried to explain the situation.

'I'm on my way,' he said.

She was in exactly the same position when I returned: still staring blindly ahead.

'Angela, tell me what's wrong. Who was that man? Is he your husband, perhaps?'

She nodded. 'He's found me. I can't stay – I can't.' She

struggled up again, but I pushed her gently back onto the settee.

'What do you mean? Has he threatened you?'

She stared at me for a moment then suddenly looked round in a panic and sniffed the air. She sank to the floor and began to twitch. Epilepsy!

At that moment, Dr Mac arrived and, taking in the situation immediately, knelt beside me and together we prevented Angela from injuring herself. Her dressing gown had slipped open and we could see bruises on her arms and legs. The result of other fits or signs of abuse?

Gradually, she quietened. She was dazed and tearful but no longer belligerent, so we got her onto the settee and tucked her up for warmth. She kept looking fearfully at the door but seemed to take comfort from having Dr Mac beside her. With gentle probing and tactful questions, he got the story out of her.

The man I had seen was her husband, whom she had left years ago when he became an alcoholic and had started to be violent towards her and her two children, now grown up. Being a Roman Catholic, she had never divorced him. She had had epilepsy nearly all her life but, like so many, was embarrassed and kept it a secret even from the Nursing Services Board that employed her.

Recently, her widowed mother had died, leaving Angela quite a large sum. Somehow the husband had heard about it and kept turning up to demand money. She kept moving and changing jobs, and she didn't know how he had found her this time.

Dr Mac was interested in the epilepsy. 'What are you on?' he asked.

She mentioned one of the latest drugs on the market: one which allowed most people to lead a normal life.

'So why the episode, then?'

'He threw the tablets away!' She burst into tears.

'So why has he gone now? And where?' I wanted to know.

'I gave him a cheque for two thousand pounds to get rid of him.' Another storm of weeping. 'I wanted that money for my daughter's wedding – now he's got it! And he's gone now.'

'Where? How?' We asked in unison.

'To the mainland. He has a motorbike hidden somewhere in the village.' She looked at us and shook her head. 'You won't catch him,' she moaned.

Dr Mac and I smiled at each other.

'Oh yes, we will, my dear,' he said. 'That husband of yours has forgotten one thing – there are no ferries on Christmas Day!'

Mr Robertson's Christmas was spent in Papavray's only police cell!

SIX

Back to work

The family had decided to wait for my return from duty before Christmas Day began in earnest. Andy was bouncing about impatiently. John and Nick and George had given up and gone for a walk, but much laughter could now be heard from the porch as they yanked each other's boots off. Beth had been ordering Paul around while she attended to the cooking. He had done a great job with the table, which looked very festive.

Thanks mainly to Beth, Christmas lunch was delicious. Later, we all relaxed in front of a blazing fire. We had coal mixed with the peat, as peat alone does not blaze in a cheerful fashion but skulks in the fireplace producing heat, blue smoke and a delightful smell but very few flames. The crofters told us it was possible, but we never managed to get our peats dry enough to do much more than smoulder.

On Boxing Day, I rang head office to explain about Nurse Robertson and to request a replacement relief nurse. There was instant consternation: there were none available. It being Christmas week, many of the district nurses had taken due leave (in many cases long overdue) to visit far distant relatives or, like myself, had family to stay. Could I manage for now, I was asked. (A rhetorical question, of course, for what was the alternative?) They would get one as fast as possible. This was a well-meant but totally unbelievable promise. So the status quo remained.

Now that Christmas was over, George had to start to earn a living on the island. Gone were the days of monthly salaries. Except mine, of course, which was quite handsome at the moment, as I would be back, once more, to working all the time.

George seemed to think that, in addition to the electrical and TV aerial work, the main source of income would come from the little boatyard, on boats that were in for refits and from the fishing fleet that put in to the harbour at weekends. To begin with, he was only considering the Papavray fleet of some dozen or so boats, but he soon found that many of the big east coasters that came among the Hebridean islands for the herring would put in to the nearest harbour if they had engine or electrical faults, or if the weather was bad.

Just before New Year, it started to snow again. My heart sank. It would not endear the captains of the boats in harbour for just the weekend if George were to be snow-bound. Quite often Saturday was the only day that any maintenance could be done on these vessels, as most of their captains were Calvinists and so forbade work on the Sabbath. The one and only bus, all shops, ferries, fishing and any kind of fun were at a standstill on the Sabbath.

There were exemptions from the 'no work' rule, which came under the rough headings of 'mercy', 'emergency' and 'necessity'. A district nurse was exempt so far as 'emergencies' were concerned, which was just as well, and 'mercy' could be made to fit almost any medical eventuality. 'Necessity' applied mainly to the feeding of livestock and the milking of cows, but human food had to be prepared on the Saturday. Things have relaxed a little over the years and the insidious apostasy blamed on incomers like ourselves.

George and I often found ourselves dealing with the same people as we went about our vastly different jobs. One day, just after the Christmas 'break', I paid one of my regular visits to an old bachelor by the name of Euan who lived in Cill Donnan. George had mentioned the old chap as being one of the first to demand a TV set and aerial. Euan was a determined customer and luckily his house was so high that there was no trouble in obtaining a signal. He was mightily impressed when George switched on the flickering picture. Later, he was to boast that he had the clearest picture on Papavray. He was not so impressed with me!

We had many old bachelors living on Papavray, as on all the Hebridean islands. This phenomenon is attributed to the lack of work, which caused so many young men to join the Merchant or Royal Navy, many giving their lives in wars and peace alike on the unforgiving sea. Living the nomadic life of seamen, they opted to remain single until they retired or were obliged to return to work the crofts on the death of their parents. To their dismay, they often found that the women had been less patient, aware that their biological clocks were ticking inexorably towards a time when they would be past childbearing. And how they all loved children! These women usually married mainlanders or the few men who remained behind.

Old Euan was one of those old sea dogs who had never found a partner. He was nicknamed 'Get Oot' by Nick and Andy, or, if I was not supposed to hear, 'Bloody Hell'.

And not without reason! Tall and shambling, he spent most

of his time in the pub. There were only two on the island and his house was almost next door to one of them. When roaring drunk, Euan deeply resented the summer tourists who often sat in the sun on the wooden benches against the pub wall. On wobbling out of the door, screwing his eyes up in the bright light, he would scowl horribly at these unfortunate folk and bellow, 'Bloody hell, get oot o' here!' They usually did!

This morning, the smell that wafted from his open croft house door as I approached was redolent of unwashed clothes, old dogs, mice and something else that I didn't even try to identify. He was sitting by the fire in his wellies, staring at the blank screen of his bright new 'teleeffission' as though awaiting the first glimmer of the evening programmes.

Hanging from a hook over the smouldering peats was an old-fashioned iron saucepan from which bubbled some malodorous pink froth that was running down into the fire.

'What on earth is that, Euan?'

'This? Tis me dinner, Nurse.'

I gazed at the disgusting mess that fizzed and spluttered as it reached the hot peats.

'But what is it?' I asked in horror.

'Ach. Tis sheep's lungs. Old Ben and Gyp are going to have some too.'

I gulped and hastily turned my attention to the reason for my visit.

'How's the sore leg today?'

'I dinna know how it is. I canna see it, can I?' he replied grumpily.

'What do you mean?'

'Well, I canna see through ma boots and I canna get them off!'

I stared at him.

'Euan, you can't mean that you have not had your wellies off since I was last here?'

'Aye.'

'But what about at night?'

'I slept in them o' course. What would I do else? Four days and nights I've had these boots on.' There was a note of pride in the old fellow's voice.

I have often wished that, just as one can close one's mouth and eyes, noses had some similar mechanism so that smells, such as the one I knew I was about to encounter, could be avoided.

'I'm going to have to remove these boots, Euan. I might have to cut them off.'

'You canna do that, Nurse! These are ma only boots! I have no more to me.'

His protests were in vain. I tried to get those wretched boots off as gently as possible, but with every tug he bellowed in pain, so I was forced to cut them off. Both of them. Although the ulcer was on the right leg, I knew that four days of incarceration in a rubber boot (held cosily near the fire) would undoubtedly have caused the ulceration of the varicose veins in the left as well. And it had.

'Thems was good, good boots,' he kept moaning. 'How am I to get more, Nurse?'

'With legs like these, you won't be going out for a while anyway, Euan.'

I was wrong. I continued to dress the legs for several weeks while, with dogged persistence, Euan plodded to the pub every day in a pair of ancient slippers!

There was another old seaman whom George and I saw in

our different capacities almost daily. He lived near the steamer pier and, in the manner of many old sea dogs, spent all his time watching the inter-island steamer coming and going and chatting to the tourists. To old Angus, smart modern cars were a source of wonder.

One day, a disembarking passenger in a very streamlined vehicle asked him how far it was to Cill Donnan.

Glancing admiringly at the sleek monster, Angus replied, 'Ach, tis five miles but in that you'll do it in three.'

On another occasion, when it was announced that the outgoing steamer would be 30 minutes late departing, an impatient visitor was complaining loud and long until Angus got tired of his grumbles.

'Ach, haud your wheesht, man. It'll no take you long to wait half an hour!'

Celtic logic, perhaps?

SEVEN

A castle and a corpus

So Hogmanay approached. I was not looking forward to the usual crop of casualties, many of them self-inflicted by over-indulgence, and the snow would be an added complication.

The crofters did not start their celebrations in earnest until midnight, when the men would grasp their bottles and visit every house in their village and those with transport might venture farther – even if the 'transport' was an ancient tractor. The very old and the very young and the women folk would stay at home to receive the revellers, the women having baked cakes and pies, boiled clootie dumpling and made Scotch pancakes 'to keep out the cold' (and to soak up the whisky, no doubt). The occupant of each home visited was required to take a dram from the caller's bottle. The caller would then graciously accept the same amount, or more, from the bottle on the sideboard. As the night wore on, the steps became wobblier, the drams bigger and the visits longer until some of the merrymakers were overcome by sleep. Usually in someone else's house.

Being unable to keep up with this rate of consumption, Beth and I, as the women of the house, and therefore left behind to receive these characters, had a 'system'. We courteously accepted the drams (one each) and pretended to sip them, saying that we were used to drinking slowly (unlike the locals who 'downed in one'), gave the expected dram in return and, after the visitor had departed, took the contents of our glasses, which had not actually touched our lips, and poured them into the bottle on the sideboard ready for the next caller. As all the crofters seemed to favour the same well-known brand, the mixture was quite acceptable. At the end of the night, we had more whisky than when it started!

Meanwhile, the men of our household roamed from house to house with their bottles, handed out the required amounts, actually drank very little but ate a great deal. George always said that Mary's clootie dumpling was excellent and why wasn't mine nearly so good? My reply is unprintable!

On this particular Hogmanay, all the family had been asked to the laird's home for early evening drinks. Duncan and his family lived in Dun Ruadh, a small castle of ancient origin. It had been in ruins when Duncan's father had become clan chieftain, and he had renovated about half of the building and stabilised the rest as an attractive ruin.

We entered by a huge oak door made from timbers recovered from an old shipwreck. This led into a high-vaulted baronial hall. A blazing fire burned in an enormous granite fireplace (the coal boat had obviously called at the pier recently, as peat would never burn like that). A few prints and paintings of animals and hunting scenes adorned the walls.

Present were Dr Mac and his wife, Fiona, with her halo of very white fluffy hair. She walked with two sticks as she was arthritic: a complaint that afflicted many of our older people, probably due to the damp atmosphere of the Western Isles. Alistair, with unlit pipe firmly in place, was sitting with Alice on a high-backed wooden settle, and Richard, the factor, strode about helping Duncan. Richard was a tall ex-army Englishman. His equally tall wife, Elaine, was also English, and local gossip had it that she had been a minor film star. Her father, Sir Kenneth Somebody, sitting close to the fire, was also an ex-officer and still had a military bearing.

We were greeted effusively by Felicity, who was a superb hostess. She was a beautiful, well-groomed woman who had met Duncan when they were both at Oxford. Her father was an earl and felt that marrying a mere clan chieftain and living on a remote island was letting the family down. She didn't care. She and Duncan were very happy and had raised a noisy brood of daughters before the long-awaited heir arrived. I knew all the children well, as they were always in some sort of trouble – bruises, cuts, toothache, broken bones, a near drowning and now chickenpox.

'Ha, Mrs MacLeod! Welcome, welcome,' Duncan tended to boom.

I introduced everyone and then left Duncan and George to chat. It proved to be one of the most lucrative 'chats' of George's life. The laird wanted the entire castle wired. Electricity had not reached the Western Isles at the time of the renovation, so a noisy generator produced the lighting that we enjoyed this evening. He wanted lights everywhere, night storage heaters in every room, power for all the usual domestic appliances and three showers. He handed the whole contract to George there and then. It was a mammoth task that would keep our family for about a year.

Later, I was sitting with Elaine when I noticed her father in deep conversation with John and Nick. They were listening with rapt attention.

Elaine saw my glance and said, 'I think he's telling them one of his war stories.'

Many of us were drinking coffee by this time, and I was surprised to notice that he was drinking his from a steaming mug that he held with both hands, disregarding the handle. It did not seem to fit with his stately bearing. Later, the boys were agog with a tale that explained it and which accounted for their fascinated faces.

It seemed that Sir Kenneth had been in the RAF during the war and had been shot down over Germany. He had been captured and sent to a prison camp but had proved a great nuisance to the Germans by insisting on better conditions for the servicemen incarcerated with him. They moved him to another camp with a more brutal regime in the hope of breaking his spirit, but the strategy misfired when he and several others tunnelled their way out. Two of his colleagues were shot while he and 'the Dauphin', a French officer, were once again recaptured. The German authorities were taking no risks this time and sent them both to Colditz. Its impregnable position successfully foiled all their attempts at escape, but they spent much time in the cold, damp dungeons in solitary confinement. However, one guard was susceptible to bribery and agreed to bring Sir Kenneth one hot drink per day. Hence the hands cradling the mug. Hands that had been blue with cold and only felt blessed warmth once daily. It was a habit that had never died. Sadly, we didn't see him again for he had not escaped the bad health that these brave men so often suffered later in their lives. He died the following winter.

We went home before midnight: the men to join the ranks of the first-footers, Beth and I to await the arrival of the early and therefore more sober revellers.

A castle and a corpus

The night went without undue incident until Paul burst in at about 2 a.m. saying that, on his way home (he had had enough), he had seen a pair of wellington boots sticking out of a ditch. They had been upside down, but he could not see much as his torch had gone out.

'We'd better go and see what's happened,' I said.

Leaving Beth to cope, we set off. Flurries of snow stung our faces as we struggled across the croft. I had already guessed that it would be old Hughie. Well into his 80s, he should have stayed at home but insisted on accompanying the 'young fellows'. I was wondering how long he had been in the snow, and I was fairly sure that we were about to find a corpse – or 'corpus', as the locals termed it.

Paul led me straight to the spot and there were the boots, sole-side up, sticking out of the snow like two skyscrapers. We jumped into the ditch, sinking to our thighs in the soft whiteness. Where was the owner of these boots?

There was a shout and George and the rest of the boys arrived. As the first of them landed in the ditch, there was a moan and some very indistinct swearing from somewhere below us. Looking at each other in amazement, we all began to scrape away the snow and soon found a tweed-covered arm and a flat-capped head. Two bleary eyes gazed up at us and gradually we extricated a very cold and very angry old man.

'Where are ma boots? I had on ma boots, I'll have ye know! And I'm away to wee Morag's and I canna be going all that way wi'out ma boots.'

Young Fergus was shaking the boots free of snow, impatient to get back to the celebrations.

'We have your boots here, Hughie, but you canna wear them the now. They are full of snow. What for were you takin them off, ye daft old bodach.'

'I didna take them off, ye silly wee mannie. I was jumpin o'er the wire and I got caught up.'

The old fellow was shivering so much that his teeth (the few that he had) were chattering, and he was wet through as the snow on his clothes began to melt.

'Home with you, Hughie,' I said.

George and the boys volunteered to take him home and hand him over to his long-suffering wife. About an hour had passed when Beth and I heard laughter and the family came in, cold but well fed and full of some great joke.

'You'd never guess. We took Hughie home and Dolleen bundled him inside. We went to two more houses and then started to walk home. We couldn't believe our eyes when we saw Hughie out and about again. He was on his way to wee Morag's in his socks!'

EIGHT

Deep ditches and high hills

The winter snows and Hogmanay celebrations had not finished with me yet. On the morning of New Year's Day, the village was slumbering in the silver/blue dawn as everyone slept off the effects of the previous night's jollifications, and I knew that folk on 'the other side' would be in a similar comatose condition. I was unlikely to hear any news about the state of the hill at Loch Annan, so I would just have to hope that I could make it to my regular visits.

So off I went: a lone little car on the narrow rutted road on the first day of 1971. With a few sideways waltzes and some tyre spinning, I was soon over the top and on my way to Cill Donnan. I attended to my first patient, a diabetic, and set off for the second.

As I approached the croft house, the usual three large dogs of indeterminate ancestry came rushing towards me, chorusing their disapproval of my intrusion. Bringing my trusty rolled and pointed umbrella into play, I waved it in a threatening arc before me and the dogs retreated, still creating a fearful din. Only once did a dog oppose this lethal-looking weapon and then he bit the point right off!

The deafening noise was further amplified this morning by

Katherine, who came hurrying towards me, shouting at the top of her considerable voice. I could not understand a word that she was saying, so she turned her attention to quieting the dogs by means of more yelling. Finally, they slunk away and blessed peace reigned.

'What on earth is the matter, Kate?'

'Nurse,' she puffed, out of breath from her efforts. 'You've to go to Dr Mac's. Y'see, I sent wee Geordie to the doctor to see would he get something for his dad's sore head. The poor mannie does suffer so . . .' She paused for want of breath.

Privately, I thought that the 'sore head' probably had a lot to do with the aftermath of Hogmanay rather than any medical condition.

'Dr Mac said when you come to do Granny, would you go to see him,' she continued with importance.

'GEORDIE!' she bellowed, attempting to attract her son's attention. He emerged from the byre.

'Do you know what's wrong, Geordie?' I asked, in a more moderate tone. Contrary to his mother's apparent belief that her son was deaf, Geordie's hearing was quite normal. I think he was so used to being yelled at that he just didn't bother to reply until his mother did yell!

'Old Charlie's in bother. It's the drink, I think,' he said in unconscious rhyme.

Nothing sounded too urgent. If I knew anything about Charlie, he'd be in the throes of a bout of DTs again. Reassured, I went into the house to my patient.

Florence McClellan was about 80 years old and was one of my patients who spoke very little English. Unlike her gargantuan daughter, my patient was a frail and gentle lady, much given to sitting too close to the fire because someone

58

was always leaving the door open and she could never get warm. Unfortunately, this habit gave rise to numerous leg ulcers that needed constant attention.

Having applied new dressings, I faced the wrath of the dogs once more and made my way to see Dr Mac. As there was no surgery on New Year's Day, I went straight to his home. The house was set in a tiny wood near the steamer ferry at Dalhavaig and on sunny summer days it appeared idyllic in its sylvan surroundings. In winter, however, it was dark and damp with tortured trees reaching starkly skywards to throw black shadows on the house. Dr Mac and Fiona had lived in the draughty old place for 40 years in perfect contentment and appeared not to notice its shortcomings.

Fiona came to the door in answer to the clanging of the old-fashioned bell.

'Come in, come in, Mary-J. A Happy New Year to you!' Although often in pain, she was always cheerful and now gave me a lovely smile as I returned her greeting.

'Himself is in the study. You know the way,' she said.

After the usual greetings, Dr Mac told me about Charlie's latest escapade. Charlie Two (why the 'Two' I have no idea) was a roadman. All over the Highlands and Western Islands, there is an indispensable body of men called 'the Roadmen'. Weatherbeaten and hardy, these men work alone on their allotted stretch of road, sometimes as long as 20 miles. They are employed to dig and clear out the fast-flowing ditches at the sides of the single-track roads and generally keep these vital links between remote villages open. On my rounds, I would see these stalwarts trudging along, shovel and spade over their shoulders, in all winds and weathers.

Charlie Two was a wiry 60 year old, always ready with a

cheery wave. But it seemed that this Hogmanay had been just one more example of his tendency to go on periodic and colossal binges. For months, he would be the model crofter and roadman, and then, for some reason that no one could fathom, he would be off again. He would neglect his work, his croft and himself. But never his dog! No matter how Charlie forgot everything else, Joc was never without a meal or a fuss and appeared to be quite content to spend long hours lying quietly under a barstool.

There was a twinkle in Dr Mac's eye as he began to tell me about the old man's latest adventure.

'Charlie had apparently been wishing everyone a "Guid New Year" all night. When he finally set out for home, the snow was very deep and he was most unsteady on his feet . . .'

'And he fell into a ditch,' I finished for him. What was the matter with everyone this Hogmanay? First Hughie, now Charlie.

Dr Mac laughed, 'Aye, he did indeed. A good deep one of his own digging.' He became serious. 'If it had not been for that dear old dog, Charlie would probably be dead.'

Evidently Joc had barked and howled and scrabbled at the snow but been unable to rouse him, so the intelligent animal finally ran to a nearby house and scratched at the door.

'My door,' said Dr Mac, shaking his head in wonder. 'Did that dog know that he had chosen one of the very few houses where the occupants were sober?'

'And he led you back to Charlie?'

'He did, and I got the old fellow out. What a state . . .' He shook his head again.

It has to be said that this so-called 'old fellow' was probably a good ten years Dr Mac's junior! In spite of his advancing years, however, the doctor had managed to drag the inert form back to his house, where he and Fiona had warmed and revived him. Later, with much help from a startled guest, he had taken Charlie up to his croft house and put him to bed. Accompanied, of course, by Joc.

'And now,' concluded Dr Mac, 'I'd just like you to look at his cuts and grazes.'

I climbed up to the ramshackle croft house wondering how the two elderly men had managed to virtually carry Charlie up the steep slope in the darkness. I pushed open the door and called his name. Obtaining no reply, I ventured into the bedroom, where Charlie was sitting up in a grubby and rumpled bed, looking bemused. Unshaven, with hair on end, he was absent-mindedly stroking Joc, who was sitting serenely on the pillow beside him.

'Hallo, Charlie.' I felt that this was not a good time to wish him a 'Happy New Year'. 'Are you feeling better?'

With an obvious effort, he seemed to focus. He frowned. 'Nurse? What's happened? What are you doing here?'

Before I could answer, Joc barked in Charlie's ear. This seemed to chase away the remnants of the old man's near-coma.

'Ach, he's needin his breakfast.'

'Tell me where everything lives, and I'll see to it.'

'There's tins in the back. He'll need two.'

I departed to 'the back' – a kind of lean-to – and there stood dozens of tins of top-quality dog food. Finding a battered bowl, I looked around for a tin opener. There wasn't one, but beside the bowl and liberally spattered with dog meat was a murderous-looking knife of immense size. It was obvious that I was going to have to stab the tins and tear the lids off with this implement.

Joc stood beside me, patiently waving his tail gently to and fro. Finally, leaving a contented Joc munching an enormous pile of meat with the water bucket handy, I returned to Charlie.

'Nurse, I remember now. I was in the ditch, but who brought me home?'

He was very embarrassed when I told him that it had been the doctor. Charlie had great respect for Dr Mac, who had treated him for many a bout of DTs over the years. But as I explained that Joc was the real hero of the night, tears came into his eyes, and when the dog reappeared, licking his lips, he hugged him with obvious love.

'Ach, I don't know what I'd be doin wi'out him, Nurse.'

'You'd be pushing up the daisies. That's what you'd be doing, Charlie! You'll have to ease up on the whisky, you know.'

'Aye, I will, Nurse, I will.'

Hmm! Until next time, I thought.

At that moment, Mary-Ann bustled in, kicking the snow from her boots. Joc greeted her with ecstasy.

'Now, what's the silly old bodach been up to this time?' was her cheery greeting. 'And how's the wee boy, Nurse?' she continued. Andy was always referred to in this way, and I wondered how tall he would have to grow before he was no longer this 'wee boy'.

She remarked, 'The snow's coming down again! I'll see to Minnie the day, Nurse. You'd best be getting home or you'll not get over Loch Annan.'

I left them to it, knowing that Charlie was in good hands. Sure enough, the snow had been falling heavily while I had been with him and now lay thickly on the ground. I decided to follow Mary-Ann's advice: leave the non-essentials and make for home.

Deep ditches and high hills

As I urged the little car up the steep, slippery road, with the wheels spinning and huge snowflakes almost obliterating my view, I soon realised that I was in trouble. I had already gone too far and too high to turn round: there was a deep ravine on one side of the narrow road and a sizeable ditch on the other. Gradually, the wheels grew tired of the struggle and spun round unavailingly, and I slithered to an unsteady halt.

The snow continued to fall heavily as I sat in my little haven and wondered what to do. It was New Year's Day. Most of the locals would be still in bed or hungover, the patient house cows awaiting a tardy milking and the old folk wondering if there was any chance of breakfast. No one would be working and certainly none would venture up here on the snowy heights of Ben Criel. I was aware of a feeling of unreality, bordering on panic, as I realised that I could be here for a very long time. It might be hours before the family missed me, thinking that I was on my rounds.

Suddenly, to my utter amazement, I heard an engine! Turning on the wipers, I couldn't believe my eyes when I saw a tractor coming towards me from the direction of Dhubaig. I was even more convinced that the cold had given me hallucinations when I recognised the driver in the jaunty cap as a young tearaway who was drunk more often than sober, never up for work in the morning and the bane of his long-suffering mother's life. Pulling to a jerky halt, this apparition leapt off the seat and trudged towards me.

'And a Guid New Year to you, Nurse!'

'Donny! What on earth are you doing here?'

'Ach. I have a new girl. She's of the Brethren in Dalhavaig. I'm off to see her the now.'

'But . . . You're sober!' I spluttered rudely.

'Aye,' replied Donny lugubriously. 'She doesna approve o' the drink.'

I couldn't believe my ears. 'Really, Donny? I mean, do you think you are suited to each other?'

'Aye. She's a bonnie wee lass and she sings like a bird,' he sighed. 'She's going to reform me,' he added, without too much conviction. He had returned to the tractor and was heaving a rope off. I came out of shock as he called me.

'Nurse, can you tie this round the front axle? I'll turn her [meaning the tractor].'

While I knelt in the snow and located the axle, which was already icing up, he revved and rattled the wheezy old tractor into place. Whistling and brushing the snow from his eyes, he hitched us up and jumped back onto his seat, shouting, 'We're away!'

We climbed the rest of the steep hill to the summit in decorous tandem, but then the steep descent past Loch Annan commenced. The little car yawed and slithered and several times caught up with the towing tractor, as I had virtually no traction on the wheels. And all the time, the yawning shape of Loch Annan gaped hungrily at the bottom of the ravine. It was entirely terrifying!

Then, all at once, we were climbing the next hill, belching black smoke and scattering white snow in contrasting plumes as we rumbled along. By the time we reached the lower ground near our village, I was shaking with fright.

Without warning, Donny suddenly stopped. Taken unaware, I put my foot on the brake, slid swiftly forward and crashed into the back of the tractor!

'Oops!' said Donny, somewhat inadequately. He disentangled us and untied the rope. He handed me my number plate, one of my headlights and several bits of bumper.

'I'll sort that for you on the morrow, Nurse. I'll be off to see wee Fiona. You'll be fine the now!'

I thanked him through chattering teeth. He turned the tractor and was gone while I drove the half mile or so home. Two dogs and two cats greeted me, while the chickens clamoured for their corn, but of the humans there was no sign and I realised with astonishment that it was only just eleven-thirty! I made myself some coffee, but I was shaking so much that I dropped the mug on the tiled floor. At least that woke them all up!

NINE

A ceilidh and a cold corner

'That was wonderful, Janet. I'm not surprised that you did so well in the Mod.'

About ten of us were crammed into Mary's living room one cold February night. Janet had just entertained us with one of the pieces she had performed so successfully back in the autumn. Rather like the Welsh Eisteddfod, the Scottish Mod gave young people a chance of recognition in their chosen field of music or poetry. Janet played the bagpipes, a difficult instrument not always appreciated in confined spaces! But she always practised outside, standing at the end of her parents' croft house on the hill. I had heard her playing on the very first day that we had set eyes on the house that was now our home. The ancient lament had come drifting across the glen, adding its sad, haunting beauty to the peaceful scene. Tonight, it was different. Janet had just played in Archie and Mary's porch and had come back in to join the ceilidh, receiving the congratulations with her shy smile. She was 12 and already held the promise of the slender loveliness to come.

I looked around at our friends and neighbours squeezed into the small room. Marion and Murdoch were huddled into a corner. Katy, in remission from the leukaemia once more and looking fitter than she had for months, had been given a fireside chair. Big Craig, Dhubaig's roadman, sat on a milking stool by the door 'to get a wee drop air'. George, Nick, Andy and I had been afforded the comparative luxury of a two-seater settee, where we tried to look comfortable. Catriona, from the Cill Donnan shop, perched on Rhuari's knee, and the frail dining chair beneath them creaked in pain. Archie was in his favourite chair that he never gave up for anyone, while Mary bustled about with dumpling and cake. Lounging against the kitchen door was Fergie, whom we had not met before. Mary introduced him as her cousin, a salesman in 'frozen foods and other combustibles'. We were fairly certain that she meant 'comestibles'. But that was Mary!

These small ceilidhs occurred almost by accident and everyone was welcome. If this one ran true to form, another eight or nine people would pack into the little room before the evening was over. It would become unbearably hot, the windows would stream with condensation and someone would eventually be forced to open the door to allow a blast of cold, damp but blessedly fresh air into the stuffy atmosphere. But, in spite of all this, Archie would continue to throw another peat onto the blazing fire at the rate of about one every ten minutes.

We had all donated something to drink, and the unsophisticated entertainment was in full swing. There would be poems, a song or two, stories and jokes (always in good taste when ladies were present) and, the most interesting thing of all to me, reminiscences about times gone by and people long dead.

Archie threw the inevitable peat on the fire and leaned back in his chair. Lucky man! Our cramped conditions allowed for only synchronised movement and the shallowest of breathing.

'Well, Mary-J,' he said, glancing around. Archie was about the only crofter who called me anything but 'Nurse'. 'I never told you about old Morag when you bought the house, did I?'

Surprised, I said, 'No, Archie, you didn't.'

'Well, I'll tell you now if you like.'

We did like! We had always heard that there was some sinister reason for the cold spot that persisted under the stairs in spite of all the heat we put into the rebuilt and refurbished house. Until this minute, everyone had been evasive whenever we mentioned this phenomenon.

'Aye, well. It was like this, y'see,' began Archie. 'Morag was an old besom. I mind as a wee boy I was afeart of her, but as we grew, we lads used to play tricks on her. One evening, we climbed the roof and stuffed some sacks in the chimney. Then we hid and watched. Out she came, bawlin and hollerin and screamin blue murder and black as a sweep she was. By! That woman's language!' He shook his head in mock horror, as island women rarely swore. Then he became serious.

'Even as a wee girl, she was evil. She'd steal folk's cats and string them up in her byre and then invite them in to see the poor dead things. Once, when the laird, Duncan's grandfather y'understand, was ridin his lovely white horse near the castle, she jumped out, screechin and screamin, and scared the poor brute that much he threw the laird off. He broke his shoulder and the horse bolted and fell in the sea. When she grew up, she'd tramp the hills, gatherin all manner of weird plants and insects, and then she'd boil them up in a big old pot. By! Did it stink! Then when the tinkers came, she'd get them to buy it, tellin them it was medicine.'

Mary eagerly joined in, 'You mind what she did to Roddy's mother?'

'Aye, she took all the blankets off the bushes where they were dryin and threw them in the sea. Then she goes into the byre, gets the cow and drives the poor beast over the cliff. She got worse and worse, and nobody felt safe from her. She let on she had "powers". Witch's powers, y' know.'

Archie sighed, and we sensed a change of atmosphere in the room.

'Douggy's mother, Mairie, gave birth to a wee girl.'

'Ah, the soul,' put in Marion, shaking her head. Douggy, who had just come in, nodded sadly.

We were riveted. 'What happened?' asked Nick.

'That besom turned up and made all sorts of weird noises beside the two o' them and threw some of that filthy muck of hers over the child. Then she pretended to make a curse on her. Mairie screamed, but Morag just laughed and said, "That child will be dead within a week." And she was!'

Marion and Mary were openly sobbing now, although they must have heard the tale a hundred times. We were horrified.

'How?' I whispered.

Archie shook his head. 'Twas 30-odd year ago, Mary-J. Nobody knew why the wee girl went, but from the day she was born, she was dyin. She just faded away. And that wicked woman was in the kirk yard when they buried the wee soul, and she laughed and yelled that it proved that she had "the powers".'

Another peat went on the fire. Archie cheered up a little and grinned at Douggy. 'A couple of nights later, someone set fire to her byre where she kept all her potions and rubbish.'

'Aye, twas my father. Everybody knew, but no one ever spoke of it.' Douggy gave his gentle smile.

Archie resumed, 'After that, she started to get letters threatenin to burn her house down as well . . .'

'That wasn't my father.'

'I know, Douggy, but it frightened her and she disappeared for years. Nobody knows to this day where she went, but one day, back she came, even battier than ever! She'd have been about in her 50s by then, I'm thinkin. That's when we boys used to play tricks on her, and our parents never stopped us; they couldn't forgive her for all her evil deeds, y'see. Well, next thing was, some years later, her aunt turns up to look after her. Morag was too batty to be able to see to herself, y'see, and folks didna know what she might get up to. Old Shona had a job, to be sure, but she managed pretty well. She'd lock Morag up when she got too violent, and we'd hear that besom's screamin and swearin across the glen, just. Shona was a big, strong woman, very dour, and wouldn't let anyone help her. That went on for years.'

Archie took a large swig of whisky.

'Why didn't she get sent away to Craiglan?' I asked, mentioning the area's psychiatric institution.

'Ach. Too proud was Shona. She was from Uist, y'see.'

This was obviously meant to explain everything.

Having fortified himself, Archie settled back once more, Mary's face took on its rapt expression and we realised that the story was far from over.

'One night, there was even more yellin and screamin than usual, and in the morning there was nae smoke comin from the chimney. Several of us men went over to see what was the matter. My dear Lord! What a sight! The pair of them slept on that old box-bed, and that's where they were – dead as door nails! There was an old kitchen knife on the floor by the bed and blood everywhere!'

We gasped. Andy and Nick were enthralled.

'We went for the doctor and the polis and the undertaker,

and then we thought maybe we should get the minister. Well, the doctor was on Rhuna, the polis had to send for detectives and there was no money for the undertaker, so he went home again. The minister thought Shona had killed Morag and then herself, and the doctor said Morag had murdered Shona and then done away with herself. At first, the polis agreed with the minister, so the doctor wouldn't sign the death certificates. What a do that was! In the end, the polis said the doctor was right after all, and so he signed. The minister wasn't convinced and said how would he know which one to bury in hallowed ground? And he refused to bury either of them in the kirk yard. There was no family to protest, y'see, so they were buried just over the kirk yard wall. But there was no money . . .'

'They died intesticle,' said Mary importantly.

There was dead silence. I stared hard at Nick, willing him not to laugh.

Suppressing a snigger, Douggy said, 'I think you mean "intestate".'

Completely at ease, Mary murmured, 'Oh aye.'

'How long ago was all this?' asked George.

'The deaths? Oh, about seven, eight year ago. It was the year we got the hay in before August, I mind.'

'Yes, and wee Janet started school,' said Katy, smiling at a rather white-faced Janet.

'Shona didna rest easy, though. She was seen.' Mary was following a thought of her own. She nudged Archie, 'You haven't told them about the ghost.'

So there was still more?

'Ach twas only once or twice. Old Hughie thought he saw Shona walkin the hills, but it might have been the drink, and Murdoch here thought he saw her over the croft one day.'

'No "thought" about it. I did see her. Twas broad daylight and I'd not had a drink at all.' Murdoch sounded indignant.

Marion rushed to the rescue, 'Well, anyway, we told the minister and he came over to the house . . .'

'And he did an exercise,' said Mary.

'Exorcism!' Laughing, Fergie spoke for the first time.

'Aye, he did, and she was not seen again. Then he blessed the house itself, as it had seen so much evil, he said.'

Big Craig spoke up. 'Aye, but we all felt it was not fair on Shona not to be buried in the kirk yard. Just because she didna go to the kirk didna mean she was not a good woman. By! There's not many as would look after such a one for nigh on twenty years!' There were murmurs of assent. He continued, 'We reckoned she'd been tryin to tell us that she was not at peace, so some of us made a wooden cross with some wood from the shore and set it up on Shona's grave. Grand, it looked. The minister didn't like it at all, but he couldn't very well go pulling up the Lord's Cross now, could he?' He paused and then, with a sly grin, he said, 'Anyway, we buried the bottom so deep he couldn't have got it out. We all felt better about her after that.' He looked round for confirmation.

Everyone nodded, 'Aye, we did, we did.'

'I wonder why we still have this cold spot where the bed was?' asked George.

Katy spoke again. 'I think the house needs the warmth of people and laughter and love to get rid of that. It's not real cold. It's just a memory. A memory that will fade now that you are here and your family comes and goes, and good things happen. The house does not have any evil there any more, so it will forget all the dreadful things.' She stopped and looked round. We were all staring at her. She blushed and we looked at the fire instead.

I had the oddest feeling, as though I were listening to someone who knew so much because she was close to knowing everything. In other words, close to death – the ultimate knowledge. Lovely brave Katy, who looked so well at the moment. Was this remission to be short-lived? I was suddenly very sad.

George was speaking. 'What a tale! And you were all involved.'

'Aye, we were, we were.' Again, the older ones nodded in unison. Then, by some unacknowledged resolve, the subject was changed, while dumpling, Scotch pancakes and tea were handed round.

When we wandered homewards across Archie's croft, the sky had cleared to a crispness that dispelled the heat and smog of cigarettes and peat smoke, and we took in lungfuls of clean air.

'Mum. Look!'

We looked skyward. All around us were shimmering curtains of gold and blue and red, flowing to and fro like the swishing drapes of an opulent theatre stage. We turned slowly through 360 degrees and the same lights were above, to the sides, behind – everywhere at once! Like a huge domed tent of some fabulous, golden fabric, the northern lights displayed their splendour in a beautiful, swaying, rhythmic movement that glittered and glowed in the night sky. Awed and amazed, we could only stand and watch. I could imagine choirs of angels, jewelled harps, Heaven's golden gates and, perhaps, God himself, walking in the billowing space surrounded by these magnificent lights. I could only wonder at the marvels of this universe and the diminution of puny humanity when faced with such grandeur. Scientists can explain the aurora borealis if they wish, but they cannot take away its impact on an individual's consciousness. What we know and what we feel do not always coincide. I have seen the 'Merry Dancers' many times since but never in such splendour as on that night, and it is an experience that will remain with me for ever.

TEN

Flora and Annie

One very cold morning, I woke at about 5 a.m. I lay in the warmth of my bed, thinking how lucky we were and how warm and cosy the house was in spite of the freezing weather outside.

I was brought back to earth by the phone. Oh no! When a district nurse's phone rings so early, it usually means trouble. It was the doctor.

'I apologise for ringing so early, Nurse. Loch Annan is impassable at the moment, I'm afraid, so I can't get to your side of the island. Rather a nasty spell of weather,' he added in his precise way.

Dr MacDonald, or Dr Mac as the patients always called him, was something of an anachronism with his old-fashioned ways, immaculate appearance in rain, wind, snow or hail and his gentle way of understating everything. He was the sort of man who might refer to the Second World War as 'an unpleasantness'. However, in spite of his mild manner he was often vociferous in his condemnation of Free Kirk dogma as expressed by some of the clergy. Far from being intimidated by his almost Victorian bearing, the patients loved him. I think he was a link with a past that may not have been good but at least they understood it. Life was moving too fast for many of them now.

'I've had a message, via the postman, from Annie-Mac in Glen Muic about her sister. Flora's tranquillisers do not appear to be working too well and she is becoming quite violent. She needs a visit and if you have anything that would . . .'

We went off into a discussion about drugs as I tried to drag on a dressing gown whilst holding the phone under my chin. I rummaged in my bag. Yes, I had the necessary drug, which would have to be given by injection.

'Annie-Mac herself may need your help too. Apparently Flora has bitten her arm.'

'Is young Angus at home just now?' I asked. 'Young' Angus was probably a lot older than I was, but in keeping with tradition he had been given the same name as his father, so the 'young' had been added to identify him and it had stuck into middle age.

'No. He is at sea. May I suggest that you take a helper with you? Let me know how you get on.'

I knew that I would probably find the old lady naked. She always stripped off when she had one of her little 'spells', as her saint of a sister called these outbursts, but I didn't have time to rouse one of the crofter women, especially so early, so it would have to be George. A very startled and wary George was woken and given a brief rundown on the situation, the need for speed and for strength, which was why he was coming.

Leaving a quiet and sleeping house, we set off along the coastal road to the track, about three miles away, which led into a wild valley. 'Glen Muic' meant 'valley of the pigs', so I suppose that at some time in the past pigs must have been kept on the island, but I never met anyone who remembered. The track soon petered out and we had to finish the journey on foot. Of course it was raining!

The house, high on the hillside, was really no more than a wooden shack: a hotchpotch that had started life as a sheiling, a rough dwelling crofters used while grazing their sheep high in the hills in the summer months. It had been extended and 'improved' but was still a poor place for two old ladies. There was no smoke coming from the chimney.

As we approached the door, Annie's querulous voice bade us 'Come away in.' She was calling from the only bedroom, just off the tiny hallway. George hung back as I entered the cold, smelly room. On the floor by the bed lay the huge, naked figure of old Flora. A face flannel, or something like it, had been stuffed into her mouth, presumably to stop further biting with her few remaining teeth. Sitting astride her middle, wearing a thick coat and gloves, was Annie – Annie-Mac to all. She was trying to keep a blanket on her screaming, thrashing sister. Poor Annie! Flora had developed dementia about four years ago and Annie, a widow for many years, considered it her duty to look after her. It was too much for her, though, and when Flora had these violent moods, she was in real danger.

'Oh, Nurse. I'm that glad you're here. I didna know if postie would remember to tell the doctor.'

'Postie', from the Royal Mail, came only twice weekly, the last visit being the previous evening. He was Annie's only contact with the outside world.

Kneeling beside them, I asked, 'How long has she been like this?'

'Two, maybe three days.'

Annie had a bloodstained hankie round her arm. The blood was congealed and dark.

'When did that happen?'

'Day afore yesterday.' And with that Annie fainted!

Quickly moving her to one side, I called to George.

'Cover Flora up,' I ordered.

'What? She's naked!'

'Yes. Just do it, please.'

He pulled some of the blankets from the bed onto the still-screaming old woman. I delved into my bag and quickly drew up the maximum permitted dose of tranquilliser, as advised by the doctor on the telephone. I had to hold the arm with a grip like a vice to keep her still.

'Hold her down for a few more minutes. I have to see to Annie.'

With no trouble, I was able to lift her slight weight onto the only bed, which the two old ladies must have shared (and Flora would undoubtedly have been incontinent). I pinched the skin on Annie's arm, finding that she was badly dehydrated. Rubbing her hands and feet brought her round, and in a panic she tried to sit up.

'Lie still, Annie. Flora's quiet now. We'll see to everything.'

I relieved George so that he could go and find water and some way of heating it to make Annie some tea. The kitchen fire had obviously been out for days, so George lit the old Primus stove.

We managed to dress Flora in a voluminous nightie and then we began the formidable task of lifting her 20 or so stone off the floor and onto the high old-fashioned bed. We pushed and pulled, first her top half and then one leg and then the other. As fast as we got one piece of her on the soft feather mattress, so another part fell off. There didn't seem to be anything firm to hold. Finally, however, she was there and by that time almost unconscious. The tranquilliser had done its job.

George brought in a cup of sweet tea. All the strength that Annie had had to muster to deal with Flora had now gone, and I had to support her so that she could drink. With the rest of the hot water, I bathed the deep tooth marks on her arm.

George found some sticks and then some rather damp peat and managed to light a fire in the bedroom while I rummaged among the oddments of food on the kitchen table (there was no larder or cupboard). I found some oatmeal and made a little slightly lumpy porridge on the Primus stove. I spooned this into Annie's mouth. At least we could get food and drink into Annie, but Flora, too, in spite of her leviathan proportions, was dehydrated and probably had had very little or nothing to eat for several days.

Annie dozed; Flora snored. George and I sat in the kitchen. Young Angus would have to be informed, of course, but we had to do something now. Flora would not be 'out' for more than about four hours and neither lady could be left here.

I looked round. Stone floors, rotting wooden walls with tendrils of fungus growing up them, a vast old range, a few pots and pans and bits of crockery. A table, three chairs and an old couch, presumably where Angus slept when at home, completed this sad home. No electricity, no water and no sanitation bar a bucket in a little shed out back. How could Angus leave two old souls in a place like this? But they did, these seamen for whom the sea was everything.

'We can't get an ambulance over as Loch Annan is still blocked,' I muttered.

Sometimes we took patients out by sea, but we were high on a hill here and a long way from the sea: even farther from any harbour or jetty.

George grinned, 'Well, it's the helicopter again, isn't it?'

He was right, for I could see no other way.

'I'll have to stay here. You go home and ring the doctor. He can get the RAF this time.' I wrote a quick note for George to dictate over the phone.

Off he went and I looked about outside. I was relieved to see that the helicopter should be able to land fairly near to the house. The weather did not look good, but there was no wind, so I hoped they would consider this to be a 'weather window'. I gathered all the old papers that I could find, screwed them up and left them, together with the can of paraffin, beside the door so that at the last minute we could take them outside and try to make a brief blaze to attract the pilot's attention.

I checked on the two women from time to time and looked about for some clothes and toiletries to pack for them, but there was pitifully little. I included a picture of Annie's long-dead husband and one of Young Angus. Now, there was a man with whom I would have words!

At last George was back, bringing reinforcements in the shape of Archie and Mary. Mary sat rubbing Annie's cold hands and feet. 'Ach! The poor soul! She's hypodermic, isn't she? She's awful cold.'

Archie just sighed and raised an eyebrow.

Dr Mac had arranged for the helicopter, which, 'weather permitting', would be here in about an hour from his call – about 15 minutes from now.

'Listen! That's the hovercopter,' said Mary.

Archie dashed outside with the bundle of paper, which he

flung on the ground. Grabbing the can of paraffin from George, he threw about half its contents onto the makeshift bonfire. We all leapt back as he followed this with a bundle of lighted matches. There was a 'Whoomph' and we had a blaze for a moment and some smoke, which we hoped the circling pilot would see.

The helicopter landed about 20 yards from the house, and once again the engines were left on. One of the crew just picked Annie up and carried her to the helicopter; she was so light. They then turned their attention to Flora. It took the combined efforts of all the men to put her onto the stretcher and load her onto the helicopter. How easy it all looks in films!

With the sea mist and drizzle worsening, the crew boarded, lifted off and were gone. We doused the fire in the bedroom, shut the rotting door and set off home for a very late breakfast.

ELEVEN

Jaynie's baby

It was a cold, crisp Monday morning as I backed my little car up the steep track from our home. The glen was white with frost, the sky a uniform turquoise, while the sea, for once blessedly peaceful, was lapping gently at the pebbly beach and eddying noiselessly into the caves on Dhubaig's shore. A winter wonderland indeed!

On such a beautiful day as this, the crofters would take time away from their chores and dawdle a little, faces held up to the unexpected sunshine, enjoying the enshrouding silence and the freedom from the usually tyrannical wind and drenching rain. They would talk of their childhood winters, which they remembered as being crisp and dry with snow for sledging and ice for skating all winter long. How we all like to linger on the stage of memories! Memories romanticised by hindsight and comforting because of it.

I was on my way to a humble abode near the pier at Dalhavaig. I had had a weird message from Ina, a crofter's wife. Ina had managed to raise seven children in her tiny house, most of whom were now grown and had left for jobs or college.

Ina would have been phoning from the post office, and she knew that Maggie, the postmistress, had sharp hearing and a lively interest in her fellow islanders, so Ina almost whispered her message.

'Nurse, will you come over here quick and don't say a word to a soul?' This was most intriguing!

As I pulled up near Ina's home by the harbour a curtain twitched and the door opened just far enough for me to sidle in. Then, to my amazement, Ina bolted it! Doors were never locked or bolted on Papavray. In fact, they were rarely shut, even in cold weather.

Ina was pale and distressed. 'Come you in here, Nurse,' she said.

I followed her into the kitchen, the usual multi-purpose room with a box-bed against the back wall. The curtains that gave this bed a little much-needed privacy were partially drawn, and I could see Ina's youngest daughter, Jaynie, a girl of about 16 or so, lying in the bed. She was flushed and upset, and failed to answer my greeting. I looked enquiringly at Ina and, without a word, she lifted the sheet. There, snuggled beside the girl, was a pink newborn baby!

For a moment, I was speechless.

'How long ago was the child born, Ina?' I asked eventually.

'Just about an hour gone. Angus was away to his work, the Lord be praised!'

Putting all curiosity aside, I spent the next 30 minutes or so doing all that was needed for mother and baby. The child was breathing well, perfectly formed and grunted gently when I picked her up. She was wrapped in one of Ina's old nightdresses. I turned my attention to Jaynie while Ina ran about collecting towels and hot water. Apart from a very normal exhaustion, Jaynie seemed remarkably well, although she was dazed and frightened.

Jaynie's baby

A few things were worrying me. The baby was quite tiny (barely 5lb, I thought) and seemed to be slightly premature. I was also becoming increasingly convinced that Jaynie was not 16. Her body was childish and unformed, and her whole attitude was immature. It was almost as if she hoped the whole thing would go away. She did not want to look at the baby, much less hold her.

Eventually, we installed the baby in a drawer, which Ina had placed beside the box-bed. I started to tell her that I would get the doctor to have a look at mother and baby later when she put her finger to her lips and made signs to me to accompany her.

'Come you into the room, Nurse.'

I followed the older woman into the adjoining room. 'Now, Ina. Tell me all before I go to get Dr Mac. Why did no one tell me that Jaynie was pregnant? No matter what the circumstances, she should have been having antenatal care.'

Ina burst into tears. 'Nurse,' she sobbed, 'you'll no believe me, but I didna know that she was expectin at all. Me! Me, as has had seven bairns to myself! And what will I tell Angus? Oh, dear, dear, dear!'

She was distraught. It looked as though she had kept her head during the last few hectic hours, but it had all been a great shock and now she was on the verge of hysteria.

'Ina, stop blaming yourself and just try to tell me how all this happened. How did she keep such a thing a secret? It seems almost impossible in a small house like this, with everyone around.'

'Nurse, I swear to you, the Lord spare me, that I knew nothin until this morning. She waited until she heard Angus goin and then she came down the stair and lay on the couch. I found her when I came in from the chickens. She had been in labour most of the night, but didn't dare let on until Angus was away.' She paused, gasping.

'Jaynie is our youngest and the only wee girl. Angus just dotes on her. He'll be beside himself, he will. Oh, he will! And he'll blame me.' Another storm of weeping followed.

I put my arm around her. What a shock she had had.

'Let's not worry about Angus just now, Ina. What happened when you found her on the couch?'

'I didna realise at first. I thought she was just puttin on so as to get off school. Then I looked at her properly and I could see that she was in labour. Oh my, my, Nurse! I was never so shocked! How could I not have seen before? I just can't take it in. Well, I'd no time to get you or anyone, because her waters went and in no time the wee soul was here. Is baby all right, Nurse? She looks awful wee.'

'I think they are both fine, for the moment, but I want Dr Mac to have a look at the baby.'

'Oh, Nurse. What will Doctor think of me?' Ina rocked to and fro.

'It isn't your fault, Ina.' I paused. 'Ina, how old is Jaynie?' She stopped rocking; she almost stopped breathing.

'Thirteen,' she whispered.

I nodded. This was worse than I thought.

'Do you know who . . .?' I got no further.

'No, I do not! But I'll murder him when I find out! May the Lord help me, so I will!'

'Jaynie hasn't said?'

'No. And I can't think who it might be. She hasn't a boyfriend and doesn't go out much. Angus always meets her after ceilidhs.'

'It must have been about last May sometime, I think. The thing is, Ina, whoever it is will be in a lot of trouble, as she is so young.'

Pre-marital sex was common among couples who were 'going together', and there were plenty of 'shotgun' weddings. But the couples were usually intending marriage anyway, so everyone, except the most pious or prudish, looked on them with indulgence. They were often very young, but not 13.

Ina had been deep in thought, and gradually a look of horror crept over her careworn face.

'Last May? Oh, the Dear Lord! No. It canna be him!' Her hand flew to her mouth and her eyes stared unseeingly across the kitchen.

'What is it?'

But Ina's eyes slid sideways as she said, 'Och . . . nothin. No, nothin at all.'

It was obvious that I was not going to get any more information on those lines, so I said gently, 'Angus will have to be told, Ina.'

She looked scared. 'No, no. Ach, he'll likely kill . . .' She stopped.

'Surely he would not harm you?'

'No, no indeed. He's a good man but . . .'

Again she stopped and seemed so distressed that I moved to the practicalities of buying or, more likely, borrowing the gallimaufry of baby equipment that would be needed.

I could do no more. The family side of all this would have to be resolved later, but for now my priority was to get Dr Mac's opinion and perhaps send Jaynie and her baby to the island hospital for a day or two.

I found Dr Mac in the middle of his surgery, and I popped

in between patients. The good doctor was virtually unshockable. He had seen much in his long career.

'Jaynie is only 13,' I reported. 'She will not name the father, but I'm sure Ina has guessed who it is and is terrified that Angus will kill him.'

Dr Mac looked at me sharply. 'She hasn't told you any more?'

I shook my head. 'It was obviously in May or thereabouts,' I mused.

'Ahh.' He thought for a moment. 'May . . . hmm.' He sighed. 'Right, Nurse. I'll be there as soon as surgery is finished. The business about the father will have to wait.'

On my rounds, I wondered about the effect of motherhood on so young a girl – physically and psychologically. That Ina would care for the baby I had no doubt, but what was this going to do to the already large family? And why was Ina so scared at the thought of the father's identity, for I was sure that she had guessed it? But I had the feeling that there was something else here. Dr Mac had reacted to 'May'; so had Ina. Why? After all, Jaynie was at school with any number of boys in May, as at any other time of the year. And how was an upstanding churchman like Angus going to take the news?

That evening, Dr Mac phoned to ask me to call in to the surgery in the morning before I went to check on Jaynie and the baby. He had an interesting tale to tell.

'I think you realised that I knew, or at least thought I knew, who the father of Jaynie's child might be. Ina realised this as well, and we had a long chat when I was there. I timed my visit to coincide with Angus getting in from his work.' He paused. 'You see, Ina and Angus had a son before they came to live here; they were in the Outer Isles then. Unfortunately, the little boy was not quite normal . . .'

With mounting horror, I realised where this was going.

Dr Mac continued, 'As he grew, he needed more care than the parents could give, as several more children had been born to them by then, so he was put into a special home on the mainland. Well, over the years his response to his treatment meant that he could be allowed out into the community – under supervision. In May of last year, his escort lost him and, to cut a long story short, he ended up here. His parents were in a predicament, as the other children had not been told about him.'

The doctor noticed my look and said with a rather sad grin, 'That is still the way of it here. Surprisingly, they had been able to keep it quiet, probably because he had been born before they came to Papavray. Well, of course, when he turned up, they had to take him in, and Angus came to me for help and advice. It was the first I had known about it all. The rest of the family were told who he was, but not Jaynie. It was still a secret from the outside world, you see, and the parents felt that Jaynie, being little more than a child, would not be able to hold her tongue. He was passed off as a visiting friend.'

Dr Mac sighed. 'It took me a while to find another place for him; we had lost all confidence in the first one. So the lad was here for most of the month of May. You know the rest.'

I was trying to take in all the implications of this appalling story. 'She is very much under age and he is her brother! What do you think will happen to him?'

'Probably nothing. He will be deemed to be of diminished responsibility and placed somewhere more secure, I would think. They might be able to keep it all out of the papers . . . I hope so for their sakes. No, he'll be all right. It's Jaynie and the baby that I'm worried about. And Ina and Angus.'

'The baby? Is the little soul normal, do you think?'

'Too early to know. We'll keep an eye on things and deal with problems as and if they arise. I'm glad that Angus and Ina are such good people. Of course, Angus is an Elder.'

I looked at him with amazement. This was Dr Mac actually praising a churchman!

'Ach well, Nurse, they are not all canting hypocrites like yon minister. There are plenty who believe in love and compassion.'

Embarrassed by expressing his feelings, he cleared his throat. 'I'll be starting the surgery now.'

But this was not the end! As Churchill said, it was only 'the end of the beginning'.

TWELVE

Bones and boats!

This particular Saturday started just like any other. Nick was home for the weekend from his school on the mainland, and he and Andy planned to take our small boat out onto the sea loch to do some fishing. We had enjoyed a spell of unusually fine weather with uncertain sunshine and a placid sea.

The boys raced about gathering fishing and boating gear, while I prepared mounds of sandwiches and thermoses of coffee. I was looking forward to a fairly light workload this morning and hoped that I would be back in Dhubaig by lunchtime. I did not quite trust the brittle sunshine and the deceptive calm. Ours was a very small boat. 'Unsinkable' supposedly, but look what happened to the *Titanic*!

So off they went and I gathered my bag and made for the door. At that moment, the phone rang.

'Nurse . . .' It was Dr Mac, and I could tell immediately that something was badly wrong. 'I've fallen and I'm sure I have fractured my leg.' He was obviously in pain.

'Fiona has called Ramsey [the ambulance] and I'm off to Rachadal, but I want you to stand in at the surgery. I'm still at home and I haven't opened up yet. Tell the patients and deal with anything you can.' He paused to catch his breath.

I was worried. Dr Mac was 70, arthritic and undoubtedly overworked. When he spoke again, he said, 'You'd better come to the hospital now, because Ramsey has just arrived. See me there and I'll give you the surgery keys, and I'll give you some numbers to ring for a locum.'

I stood for a moment, phone in hand, my mind skipping over the current patient list and trying to remember if there was much outside my sphere that day. By tomorrow we would have found a locum – I hoped!

*

'Will ye no keep still, Doctor? I canna take the pictures with you jumpin about like yon.'

The X-ray technicians were having trouble making Dr Mac sit still, as he kept shuffling notes and jotting down phone numbers.

'I'll be having a walking plaster,' announced the indomitable doctor.

'Indeed and you will not! Tis too bad a break for that. You'll no be walking anywhere for a wee whiley.'

I departed with a head full of instructions and a sheet full of the phone numbers of various retired doctors on whom Dr Mac occasionally depended.

I drove to his surgery, where a few patients were waiting, vaguely aware that something had happened to their beloved doctor. Two of them went home and two more had only minor problems that I could deal with on the spot.

I began the search for a locum, and after several abortive calls I rang a number in Glasgow. A broad Irish voice answered me.

'Dr O'Donnell here.'

I explained the situation, and he agreed to set off immediately.

'And tell that young man to mend soon!'

This was his parting shot. Dr Mac young? At 70? I wondered just how old Dr O'Donnell would turn out to be!

The weather was already deteriorating as I set off on my rounds. I was passing the harbour at Dalhavaig when I noticed a crowd gathered on the pier, which was quite a surprise as there was no steamer due for several hours. Suddenly, a figure jumped out in front of the car. I braked hard and slewed to a halt on the wet road.

'You'll get yourself killed, Shoras.'

Old Shoras, 'The Pier', squinted in at the window. 'Nurse! Young Ally's in the water!'

I stared stupidly. 'In the water?'

'Aye, he fell off the wall. He canna swim.'

I got out of the car, grabbing a blanket as I went. I followed the sprackling old man towards the agitated crowd.

There, in the murky depths of the harbour, were two figures. I instantly recognised the huge form of Rhuari, our island 'giant', striking out powerfully towards a pair of flailing arms. The watching crowd was voluble in its advice.

'Stay you still, Ally!'

'He'll sink if he does.'

'Nearly there, Rhuari!'

'Throw that life ring in, Angus.'

'There should be a rope on it.'

'Old Callum took it for his boat, the silly old bodach.'

'Throw it in anyway!'

And so on.

Meanwhile, Rhuari had reached the spluttering boy.

'Stay you still!' we heard him bellow, but Ally still struggled, grabbing Rhuari by his hair, whereupon the boy received a sharp cuff on the shoulder and was finally still. Turning him, Rhuari's spade-like hands went under Ally's arms and with a powerful kick he made for the pier. At last someone threw the lifebelt. It landed firmly on Rhuari's head!

Perhaps it was Rhuari's shock of curly hair or the giant-like proportions of his head, but he shrugged off the weighty lifebelt as though it were an annoying fly. He struck out for the steps. There he slung Ally over his shoulder and climbed to the pier.

I pushed my way through the throng to give assistance, but I was hardly needed. Rhuari upended the young lad, thumped him firmly on his back and waited for him to cough and take a good deep breath before lowering him gently to the ground. With a grin in my direction, he marched off amid much backslapping. He looked embarrassed by all the congratulations.

I wrapped the unfortunate Ally in the blanket, wiped his face and walked him to the car. He seemed no worse for his impromptu ducking, so I took him home to his mother.

Back in Dalhavaig, I did my regular visits (injections, dressings and minor childhood ailments), aware that the weather was deteriorating further, and as I made my way to Dr Mac's home I began to worry about the boys. He had insisted on being sent home, and I found him in his study before an enormous fire, with his plastered leg raised on a stool. He was drinking the inevitable cup of tea, and he looked white and strained.

I had just finished letting him know about Dr O'Donnell's imminent arrival when the phone rang. Fiona answered it and came back into the room looking worried.

Bones and boats!

'It's for you, Mary-J. Something about the boys.'

I glanced out of the window. The sea was now choppy, with huffing waves. I picked up the phone. It was 'Basher', Nick's friend from the small island of Schula. (His name was some unpronounceable Nordic word, so 'Basher' he was.)

'Mrs M! I thought you might be at the Doctor's. Nick and Andy have just landed on Isle Cruach . . .'

'Isle Cruach? Why? Are they all right?'

'Yes, I think so. I can see them through the binoculars. I was watching because I thought they were coming here, but they seem to have lost power and they have drifted onto Isle Cruach. I'd go for them, but it's too windy for the taber [his tiny boat], and Mum and Dad are on Eileen Mor with the dory.'

My head was spinning. Isle Cruach was a tiny island, only about a hundred feet in each direction. Where would they shelter?

Before I could speak, Basher continued, 'I have rung the shop that Mum and Dad were going to. They can pick Nick and Andy up on the way back. It will take about an hour or more . . .' He trailed off.

'But what if the weather worsens and they can't get back?' Even a dory would not be safe among the jagged islets in really bad weather.

'Well . . . if it holds at this, they'll get there.'

'And if it doesn't?'

'Coastguard, I suppose.'

'I'm going home,' I decided. 'Dhubaig is so much nearer. Ring me there when you know any more. Thank you, Bash.' How I hated that nickname! It suited him not at all: he was a gentle, well-mannered boy.

The blustery wind was now buffeting and shaking the little car as I made my way over Ben Criel, and the rain was so heavy that, in spite of the wipers, I could scarcely see through the windscreen.

It was getting dark now and I was becoming very concerned. George was away. I reflected irritably that he always seemed to be away when there was any family emergency. I rang Basher on Schula. (Surprisingly they had a phone on their island.)

'Any news, Basher?'

'None. I don't even know if Mum and Dad have received my message. I can't see far now it's getting so dark.'

'I think I'll ring the coastguard. There is nothing else either of us can do. Thank you, Basher.'

I was just about to make the call when there was a thundering on the back door and Archie burst in, shouting, 'Are ye there, Mary-J? Where are your boys? Your boat's no at the shore!'

He had been to secure his own boat against the storm and noticed that ours was missing. I told him what had happened and that I was about to call the coastguard.

'No good,' he said. 'Two calls already. Boats in trouble well out to sea. They'll no go for the boys if they are safe on dry land – well, not dry exactly, but you know what I'm meaning.'

I realised that he had been indulging his hobby of listening in to the emergency waveband on his old transistor radio.

'What am I to do, Archie? They won't drown, I know, but they will be cold, wet and hungry, and Andy will probably be scared.'

'I'll go!' Archie volunteered with no hesitation. 'I've a good strong boat.' He pushed his cap up and scratched his head. (This meant that Archie was pondering.) 'I'll take a crowbar and some tools so we can get into the bothy and out of the weather. Mary-J, get you some food together and blankets and something hot to drink. I'll meet you at the shore.'

He turned and was gone. I hastily boiled kettles, made thermoses of sweet tea, found some meat pies in the fridge and dumpling in the larder. I collected blankets, some towels and two eiderdowns, bundled it all into the car and made for the shore.

Archie was there already with a fearsome-looking crowbar and some elderly tools. He took the goods from me and stowed them in the small forward cabin.

'I'd like to come too, Archie, but Dr Mac is off and I . . .'

'Aye, I know. [Of course he knew. How silly of me!] And Dr O'Donnell will no get here the night in this weather!' (So he knew about Dr O'Donnell, too.)

'Fergie's comin.' Sure enough, Fergie came running down the hill, coat flapping.

We all pushed the boat down the rollers and into the heaving sea. The men jumped in and I watched until I could no longer see the masthead light that had been appearing and disappearing as the boat plunged and rolled on the tumultuous sea. I turned and drove over Ben Criel once more to see Dr Mac and open the surgery.

Fiona told me that Dr O'Donnell had phoned to say that he was stuck on the mainland. Dr Mac was asleep, so I did not disturb him. Luckily the storm had meant that most people were happy to keep their ailments until the morning, so the surgery was very quiet.

As I drove home past Loch Annan, I saw the large, muscular figure of Big Craig, our roadman, bent almost double as he battled his way towards Dhubaig and his fireside. I stopped and he climbed into the tiny car with difficulty.

'Ach! It's coarse, coarse weather, Nurse,' he grumbled, good-naturedly. 'And are your boys still on Isle Cruach?'

I stared at him in amazement. Even for Papavray's jungle telegraph, this was quick! He saw my look and chuckled. 'Murdoch was with Fergie when Archie told him, and he told Postie.'

I told him all I knew and he made me promise to 'gie him a wee knock' if I needed his help in any way.

Mary arrived. 'Will we sit together a whiley?'

We sat until the small hours, drinking tea, until Mary went at about 4 a.m. I finally fell asleep in front of the Rayburn.

'Hello, Mum!'

'Hello, Mum!'

I awoke with a start to see that it was daylight and there were my two shipwrecked mariners looking at me with wide grins on their grubby faces. With relief I saw that, although they were bedraggled and filthy, they were unharmed. Falling over each other to recount their adventures, they told me that the boat had lost power for some reason and they had drifted to the only beach on Isle Cruach. They had wisely turned the little craft upside down and crawled under it to obtain some shelter from the howling wind and horizontal rain. There they stayed for several hours, wet, cold and hungry.

When Archie and Fergie arrived, the whole thing had turned into an adventure. The bothy door was prised open, enough driftwood was gathered to make a fire, the food and blankets brought in and . . .

'I had some whisky, Mum,' announced Andy with pride.

I looked at him. 'And did you like it?'

'Um, no, it was horrible.' (He doesn't think so now!)

'I liked it,' said Nick. (He still does!)

Bones and boats!

At about 7 a.m., Fergie realised that the storm had abated, so they scrambled into Archie's boat and towed our little craft back. So here they were. Tired but feeling quite heroic. What a tale for school on Monday!

I stoked the Rayburn, made a huge breakfast, which they ate with gusto, and chased them into a hot bath. I showered, changed, fed the animals again and set off for work. Just as I shut the door, George drove down the track!

THIRTEEN

'The terrible, terrible thing'

One day towards the end of February I had a call from John, the policeman, swiftly followed by one from Dr Mac. Both were guarded and cryptic, but the three of us were to go to Chreileh, one of the smallest inhabited islands in the Hebrides. It was about three miles by two and even more remote than Papavray, as it was situated many miles farther out into the Atlantic. I had never been there.

As I drove to the steamer ferry at Dalhavaig, where I was to meet the doctor and the policemen, I puzzled over the brief message.

'Minister McDuff has called from Chreileh to say that there is a problem that needs the three of us immediately. He sounded very shaken and refused to say more, except that it concerned a neglected old lady who needed treatment and removal from the island, probably to Rachadal hospital.' This was all that the doctor had been told, and John's summons had been even less informative – just that a police presence was needed.

A small fishing boat that did winter duty as an inter-island ferry was waiting at the pier. John and Dr Mac, with his 'bag of tricks' as he called it, were already there, and we boarded immediately. We were the only passengers, as people do not travel much in the wintertime. The larger ferries do not run then, so a couple of fishing vessels are the only means of transport between the small islands.

Dougall was the owner of the *Sprite*, a pretty name for the squat, lumbering craft that smelled strongly of its primary function. Rugged and weatherbeaten like his boat, his blue jersey bespattered with fish scales, Dougall was well known to all of us. He was curious about our mission.

'I took the minister over a few hours ago,' he boomed above the noise of the engine and the howling of a force eight. The sea was rough, and we were tossed and battered as we rose onto the crests and thumped down into the troughs. The *Sprite* somehow managed to roll from side to side at the same time.

'Aye,' Dougall continued, fortissimo. 'He was prayin the whole way over. I think he's more faith when he's on the sea than he has in the kirk.'

Dougall's remark reminded me of one of George's sayings, harking back to his days in the Merchant Navy, namely that 'everyone's a Christian in a typhoon!' He had never forgotten the sight of burly stokers on their knees while a mid-Atlantic storm sent 40-foot waves over the bow of the ship. The very men who an hour or two before had been swearing, gambling, drinking and fighting!

At last we neared Chreileh and I had my first sight of the island. No pretty-pretty island this, but a stark, solitary rock rising from the vastness of the ocean. Sea girt with a restless skirt of white froth, its low hills of brown and purple slumbered beneath an angry sky full of dark scudding clouds. It looked solid: stubbornly resistant to the elements. Eternal. A testament to nature's sovereignty. The constant pounding of the cliffs and the rattling of the pebbles as the waves retreated to gather themselves for the next onslaught added another fearsome noise to the roaring of wind and rain. Suddenly, however, we were rounding a headland and entering a large bay that was comparatively calm.

The island had been home to a small whaling fleet, and the remains of the once-busy harbour could still be seen. Now it was badly silted up and there was only a narrow channel of deep water to the tiny pier. As we nosed our way in, I could see the ruins of vast sheds. Rusting roofs gaped and rattled in the wind, and bits of unidentifiable machinery stood about. The skeletons of two whalers, now half buried in the mud of the harbour, also told their sad story. Roofless houses were everywhere, while boulders and weeds littered the track leading up into the hills from the harbour. Not a tree softened the severity of the landscape, and yet there was a primitive grandeur, a glorious awareness of the forces of nature that had fashioned this little world. Only man's additions had suffered in the passage of time: the rest would go on for ever.

There was no sign of life, but we had been observed. An agitated figure rounded a far bend in the hill track and made its erratic course down to the pier as we carefully disembarked onto the slippery surface of the broken stones. A small private boat, as battered as the one that we had crossed in, was tied up alongside.

'That's Roddy's boat,' Dougall informed us. Roddy was the garage owner from Papavray who also doubled as the coal merchant and the undertaker. 'He must be here for a corpus.'

He saw my puzzled look.

'Ach, well, y'see,' he shouted. 'Folk dinna like travelling with a corpus on the ferries, so Roddy has to fetch them over in his own boat.'

I hadn't given such things much thought, but I could now see the reasoning behind Roddy's prudent decision. All the dead from the small surrounding islands were brought to Papavray for burial, so Roddy's boat afforded some privacy for the deceased and their families. This was just one more example of the undreamed-of difficulties of living in remote places, and the ingenuity of the people who did so.

The advancing minister flapped his scarecrow way along the pier to where we waited.

'May God bless us this day,' he intoned as he regained his breath. 'This is a terrible, terrible thing that has been done here.'

The Rev. McDuff was a pale, gaunt man and now the shock of whatever this 'terrible thing' was had made him look quite ill.

Dr Mac grunted. He had no time for that 'canting creature', as he was apt to call the Reverend. I suddenly realised that these two were the ones whose opposing opinions about the deaths of Morag and Shona had caused so much trouble in Dhubaig eight or nine years ago. To a feuding Gael, that is no time at all!

We followed the minister along the pier and began to ascend the track leading up the hill. Dougall tied the boat and ran to catch up, agog with curiosity. On our way, we met Roddy and an assistant coming down the hill bearing a rough wooden stretcher. On this was a rather dirty blanket, under which the shape of a body was clearly visible.

'*Ciamar a tha*' was the very subdued greeting. They did not linger but carried on towards Roddy's boat. Even these two rugged individuals looked shocked, although they were well used to the paraphernalia of death.

We tramped on past a group of houses showing signs of occupation, but there was no one about and we followed the silent black-clad minister out onto the open hillside. In the distance, we could see a larger than average house, more of a farm than a croft, and very isolated. As we approached this bleak house, we saw a knot of people near the door, whispering among themselves. What could have happened?

The minister turned to us at the door and said, 'Prepare yourselves! You will be deeply shocked.'

I stared at him and almost found myself copying his plea to God to bless us. He led us through the kitchen and up the stairs, where he opened a latch door and stood to one side. The doctor and John entered first and stopped just inside. Peering between them, I gasped in horror.

The smell was overpowering and I could see a figure huddled on a filthy bed. Dr Mac and I advanced cautiously, but John stayed back, barring the entry of Dougall and the minister. The figure was that of a woman, whose age I judged to be about 60. Her scanty clothes fell in grey rags, revealing a thin frame, while her white, tangled hair was in a kind of bird's nest at the side of her head.

I heard John move to open the window, but it had been nailed shut. The woman on the bed was looking at us with wary eyes, and her mouth was opening and closing, but no sound came. As I approached one side of the bed, I was again horrified as I saw that a length of chain was attached to the poor creature's wrist, while the other end was secured to the bedpost. Dr Mac and I looked at each other in disbelief. Was she mad? Who had done this? It looked as though she had been here for years. Some dirty plates and a jug of cloudy water stood on a grubby table near the bed, and the final degradation was in the corner of the room where some newspapers, spread on the floor, held human excrement.

Led by instinct only, the doctor and I began to murmur

soothingly. I don't think we actually said anything, just made consoling noises. She stared at us with frightened eyes.

We could hear whispers on the stairs and Roddy crept into the room and went to John. In his hand was a sturdy pair of wire cutters and a small saw.

'Chappie over the hill gave me these,' he said, nodding towards the chain.

Dr Mac pulled himself together and began to take charge. 'The first thing is clean water for her to drink and something to eat . . . maybe soup would be best. Ask a neighbour.' This was to John, who hurried off.

I needed to do something. I held out my hand to her, murmuring, *'Ciamar a tha.'*

She looked at my hand and appeared to hear my greeting, but still she said nothing. Slowly and diffidently, she touched me. I had never had to deal with anything like this before and was functioning purely on instinct and compassion as I patted her hand and gradually pressed the filthy little figure to me. She began to cry, but her weeping was strangely silent as huge tears flowed down the grimy cheeks. Not a sob or a moan.

Dr Mac stood close but said nothing, motioning to John to start cutting the chain.

I rocked the weeping woman as the sawing and cutting went on. They were afraid that they might hurt her if they cut too close, so a six-inch length of chain and the 'bracelet' had to remain for the time being.

A worried-looking crofter woman came to the bedroom door and handed me a mug of warm soup.

'Thank you,' I whispered to the kindly soul. 'Can you bring me some warm water, soap, a flannel and a towel so that I can wash her face and hands?'

I held the mug towards the woman. She grabbed it and took it in great noisy, greedy gulps. How long, I wondered, had it been since she had eaten? It seemed likely that whoever had just been carried away had been responsible for this. Who? Why? The minister was right: it was a 'terrible, terrible thing' that had been done here.

The crofter came back with the water. Indicating the figure on the bed, she whispered to me, 'Her name is Biddy.' I stared at her, but she shook her head and her eyes were wet. She was obviously deeply shocked.

I lifted Biddy's head and gently bathed her face and her claw-like hands. The dirt was unbelievable. At least I was able to address her as 'Biddy' now, and she seemed surprised to hear her name.

Dr Mac stood by helplessly, probably for the first time in his long career, and I acted only through a fog of pity and disbelief.

John motioned to Dr Mac and they went just outside the door to confer. I kept talking gently to Biddy, but, although she watched me carefully, she still made no reply.

After a while, Dr Mac came back into the room and explained that we were going to wrap her in blankets and the men would carry her down the stairs and put her on the 'stretcher' that Roddy had brought back. She would be taken to the *Sprite* and tucked up in the tiny cabin for the journey back to Papavray. She gazed at us during all this, but we still could not tell if she understood.

I began to wrap a blanket round her shoulders and another round her lower parts. It was very clear that neither her clothes nor her person had been washed for years, and my stomach heaved as I moved her.

Roddy was at the front door with the stretcher, and she was

made as cosy as possible, but that piece of equipment was not constructed for comfort, as its usual occupants were not likely to complain. The same crofter woman came forward and solicitously wrapped a waterproof coat around Biddy.

'Do you know about all this?' I asked her.

'None of us did, but we do now and can guess the reason for it . . .' She could not continue but began to shed tears of utter despair.

I looked at her. If these kindly people had not known of Biddy's plight, how must they be feeling now? To realise that this cruelty had been happening under their very noses as they went about their everyday tasks?

John came over to the little group of crofters. 'I'll be back when we have got the lady on board, to find out what you know.'

There were murmurs and sobs from the women while the men looked at their boots.

The little procession set off along the track in the blustery wind; mercifully, the rain had stopped. I walked beside the stretcher as often as the width of the path would allow and kept talking to Biddy, using her name frequently in the hope of lessening the shock of all this activity. The poor lady was very frightened.

John had contacted Papavray's ambulance and it was waiting at Dalhavaig harbour to transport Biddy, the doctor and myself to Rachadal hospital. As soon as we arrived there, my own involvement ended and I went home to bathe and wash my hair and clothes.

But all this 'washing away' of the trauma was superficial. It was days before I recovered emotionally from the horror of Biddy's plight and a week or so before I heard the whole dreadful story.

FOURTEEN

The terrible, terrible truth

'Nurse? I'm just calling to say that Chrissie is here. The lady who got the soup?'

'Yes, John.'

'I had to ask her to come over to sign statements and stuff. We wondered if you might like to hear the story from her. She's at her sister's for a few days, so you could pop in some time. Maggie, Dalhavaig post office.'

At about three the next day, I made my way to the post office as instructed. What was I about to hear?

Chrissie and Maggie, both in their late 30s, ushered me into the back room, where a bright fire and warm colours created a cameo of comfort. Maggie departed to serve a few customers.

'Oh, Chrissie. Do you know how Biddy is? I believe she is on Rhuna in Tarradon House.' This was a bright, cheerful nursing home on the neighbouring island of Rhuna.

'She's getting better. Clean, hair cut and washed, decent food and so on, but . . .' She paused and shook her head doubtfully.

'Yes, yes, I can imagine. Please tell me how all this happened. It seems so unbelievable. It's like something out of a horror story.'

Smoothing her skirt in a nervous gesture, Chrissie began a tale that could have been set in the eighteenth century, it was so unbelievable. The first thing she said astounded me.

'Biddy and I used to play together as children, and . . .'

I interrupted, 'But she's 20 years older than you!'

She shook her head sadly. 'Oh no,' she murmured. 'Biddy is 36.'

I felt cold and sick. This woman that I had taken to be in her 60s was only 36! What had those years in that dreadful room done to her?

'Please go on.'

Chrissie gave a ghost of a smile. 'Anyways, she grew up in that farmhouse. Her parents were strict Brethren, so they kept to themselves, but there was a school on the island in those days and lots more houses. The whaling was still going then, so there were about 20 families and we children had a good life. I got to know Biddy through school, and although her father was very strict her mother used to let her play with me after school. But Mairi was terrified of her dour, grim husband. We children never went near the farm if he was about, and Mairi only let Biddy come to play with me if he was away off the island for any reason.

'Biddy had two half brothers by old Donald's first wife. She died when they were only boys, but they were grown and working at the whaling by the time he married again. Mairi was not young either, and they were surprised when Biddy was born. The brothers were very jealous of her. They hadn't liked their father marrying again, y'see.

'Biddy was a pretty, dainty little thing, but not very bright. Not exactly backward, y'understand, but not good at lessons.'

Chrissie paused and sighed. 'Well, we grew from children

into young girls, and the lads began to notice us. Biddy in particular, as she was a lot prettier than I was. I started courting my Angus about then, but Donald began to keep Biddy in and wouldn't let her mix with us at all. She helped on the farm and we hardly saw her except when she came to the shop for the mails and the groceries once a week. We kept the post office, y'see. She'd linger a while, glad of the chance of some young company, I suppose. She'd chat with my brother sometimes. He worked our croft, y'see, as my father was poorly. The lass was not allowed at ceilidhs or dances. Aye, we had dances back then!' Chrissie smiled at her memories of those good days. 'Chreileh's a quiet place the now,' she added sadly.

'Well, one day after Biddy had been in the shop, I saw the two of them together on the hill where Johnny was working. Just talking, they were. But I knew! There was something about the way he was looking at her – with his head bent, you know. I was afraid for them. I knew that Donald would near break Johnny's neck if he found out that they were meeting. I spoke to Johnny about it, but what lad takes notice of his sister? Eh? He was besotted with her! She used to climb out of her bedroom window when they were all asleep and they'd meet in the byre or out on the hill, he told me.'

Chrissie sighed again. 'They were more than just friends, as you'll have guessed. But I'm sure they were very much in love. And it was time. Time for marriage! Folk married young in the islands. Still do. I was already married to Angus by then.'

She paused for a few moments and then shook her head. 'Of course, it couldn't last. Donald saw them one night when he was at a lambing on the hill. He followed them and beat them both half to death and broke both Johnny's legs. He left him there and dragged Biddy home by her hair. My father, who could scarcely breathe for his bronchitis, went out looking for Johnny and they got the poor lad off the island and to Papavray in a fishing boat. They took Johnny to the hospital, a poor little place then, not the lovely new one at Rachadal. But he never came out!' Chrissie's eyes were damp as she spoke of her brother's death.

'He got pneumonia and septicaemia, and I don't know what else, and he died after a few weeks. My father was getting worse and worse, and the shock of Johnny's death finished him too. Next thing, Donald had a stroke and died. Nobody was sorry about that death!'

She smoothed her skirt in that nervous fashion again. 'The only time we saw Biddy after that was at Donald's funeral, and she looked ill. We could see bruises on her arms and neck, but the two brothers kept hold of her so we couldn't speak. She didn't come to the shop any more. Mairi came instead and never spoke a word. Just handed over a grocery list, took the mail and the goods and went. Then Padruig and Lachy came home for good to work the farm. The whaling was done anyway. Awful men! Nobody liked them. Mean and bigoted, they were like their father before them! Just occasionally we'd catch sight of Biddy away in the distance fetching the cow or perhaps a stray sheep. Then nothing for months. One day, my mother asked Mairi if Biddy was all right and she said, "Yes, of course", but she looked kind of wary and frightened, Ma said.

'Then, about six months later, off goes Lachy to the mainland for no reason that we could see. And in their old leaky boat too. They hadn't used that boat for years. He had a big bag with him, and so we thought maybe they had had a falling out and he was leaving. I remember wishing that they had both gone, for I would have gone up there to see if Biddy was all right, but I couldna with that Padruig there and me pregnant and Angus just away to sea.

'Rumours got round that she'd gone mad, with her being a little bit simple as a child, y'see. Folk thought that Mairi was keeping her in for that reason. We know now that it wasn't Mairi's fault. Lachy had come back now and he could have turned her and Biddy out because he had inherited the farm.

'Then they started to do the shopping. Mairi was ill, they said. My mother was for calling the doctor, but they said there was no need. Well, by the time they did finally call him, it was too late. She was dead when he got there. He was a locum, so we didna get to know too much about what ailed Mairi.'

Maggie came in at this point with some tea and pulled the curtains, making the room even cosier. She had closed the post office and now sat down with us. Chrissie had a sip of tea and then continued her bleak story.

'At Mairi's funeral, we asked the brothers why Biddy was not there, and they said that she had gone away a while ago. We couldn't understand this, because no one had seen her go. On a small island like Chreileh, everyone watches comings and goings.

'Time went on and those two were only ever seen when they got a few bits of groceries and collected the mail. And there was precious little of that! But one day a letter came for them from a town on the mainland. With so few mails, my mother used to get to know people's usual letters and always noticed anything different, if you follow. Well, we thought it must be from Biddy, so we came to the conclusion that she had left after all. Maybe in their old boat again, we thought. Some years later that boat did for Padruig. He drowned.'

Another biscuit appeared to fortify Chrissie, and after a

moment she went on. 'Of course, we know now that the letter must have been from someone else or the wrong island and not for them at all. We've pieced it all together since. How could we have been so gullible? How could we not have seen what was going on?' She was weeping now, and I understood the feelings of guilt and frustration that she must have been feeling.

'You mustn't blame yourself, Chrissie. These islands are full of odd, reclusive families. Usually it's all right. Just different.'

Blowing her nose energetically, she handed Maggie her cup for a refill. She nodded but was clearly very upset.

Dreading the answer, I asked, 'So how long was Biddy a prisoner in that room, do you think?'

'Probably from the time that Mairi died, and that was in 1955.'

'Fifteen years or more! Dear God! And she'd have been . . . what? About 19, 20?'

I paused for a moment, unable to take it all in. 'And do you know now what happened to start all this?'

'Yes. John, your policeman, went through the house and found a letter that Mairi had hidden in the bottom of her sewing box. I suppose she guessed that the men would be unlikely to find it there. She wrote that she had discovered that Biddy was pregnant just after Donald died. It's as well that it was not before he died or he'd likely have killed her.'

'Lachy wanted Biddy sent away, but it would have cost him to send her to one of those places for pregnant women, and Mairi fought to keep her anyway. So she was just kept out of sight. As it happened, the men were away on one of the last of the whalings when the baby was born, so Mairi looked after him for a week or more. Biddy called him Johnny, by the way. According to Mairi's letter, she loved and nursed that baby just all the time.

'Then the men came back and immediately they decided to take the baby away. One night they just wrapped him up and Lachy went off. Oh! The cruelty and the evil of it!'

Chrissie was overcome for a moment and took a long drink of tea.

'Surely they didn't . . .' I couldn't go on with my question.

'No. Not even they were that bad. Or perhaps they just thought that they would go to hell if they killed a baby. Who knows? No. Lachy took the child to a hospital on the mainland, handed him to the night nurse on duty and ran off!

'When Biddy found that her baby had gone, she really did go out of her mind. Mairi wrote that the brothers said they had arranged an adoption. Mairi didna believe them, but they threatened to turn both women out if they tried to locate the child.

'Well, there was a lot in the letter about trying to comfort Biddy, but Mairi wasn't young and I think the whole business killed her. She had written this letter rather like a diary, and it stopped about there. Maybe she knew she was dying and that's why she hid it. When she did die, those two just shut Biddy up and treated her like an animal – or worse. Of course, Padruig drowned some years ago and Lachy just carried on by himself. He must have been 50 or more.

'Well, last week, when he hadn't turned up for the mails and we had heard the beasts bellowing because they hadna been fed and milked, we knew something was wrong, so my Angus went up there. He found Lachy dead on the kitchen floor. So he rang the minister and Roddy. He couldn't get the doctor – I don't know why. It was when the minister was praying over that Lachy (and if anybody needed prayers, it was him) that he heard a noise upstairs . . . Just think, if he hadn't, she would have starved to death up there!'

Chrissie put her head in her hands and rocked to and fro. 'If only Donald had dealt with it all decently, they could have been married before anyone knew about the baby. Johnny loved her; I know he did. He would have done the right thing. He probably had no idea that she was pregnant at the time. I don't suppose she knew herself.'

We sat in the firelit room and thought of all the wasted years and the wasted lives.

'Do we know anything about the child?' I asked after a while.

'The police have started enquiries. It will take months, I shouldn't wonder. He must be nearly a man by now – 16? He's my nephew, of course. Biddy does not seem to remember anything. Still can't walk properly. Just sort of crawls with a funny kind of hop, and she hasn't said a word. Not one! They've got psychiatrists and speech therapists and I don't know what going in to see her, but she just sits and watches people.'

Another awful thought struck me. 'Did those two beat her?'

'Doctor doesn't think so. Just put water and food into the room and removed the newspaper in the corner. They probably even thought they were doing the right thing by keeping her hidden. She was bad, you see. A baby out of wedlock. Huh! As if it doesn't happen all the time. Why, I was three months gone when Angus and I were married. No one thought a thing about it.'

We gazed at the fire in companionable grief.

Suddenly, Chrissie looked up. 'We have decided to petition to be moved off Chreileh.'

This was a surprise. I knew that the inhabitants of St Kilda had petitioned back in the 1930s and they had been relocated in Argyllshire. But there had been 20 families there. I was a little hazy about the criteria for this request to be granted, and I asked Chrissie to explain.

'I don't know if the Commission will help us. They may just expect us to make our own way because there are so few of us now: only four families and no children. We can't manage with so few men for the heavy work, and they are all getting older. We'll have to see whether they will help, but we are going anyway. This has finished us. None of us want to stay now. The men have been talking about it for some time, but if ever something was needed to make their minds up, this has done it!'

'But where would you go?'

'Probably here, to Papavray, if the men can find work. There's the forestry.'

'And the oil rigs,' added Maggie.

On that note of hope, I left them.

Biddy stayed in the nursing home for many months. I went to visit her once and she was looking reasonably fit and could walk, but there was a dull look to her eyes and she had still not uttered a word.

She was moved to a specialist home on the mainland some time in the following few weeks and remained there until her death at the age of only 41. Her heart had been irreparably damaged by the years of abuse and privation. We heard that the only time she spoke was when she saw a baby on the television.

She said, 'I had a baby.'

FIFTEEN

The wedding

One sunny day in spring, Mary came puffing over the croft in a state of great excitement. She flopped down, prepared for a good gossip. 'Have you heard about Rhuari and Catriona?'

I shook my head.

'Well, they are to be married!'

'Really?' I tried to sound surprised. 'Good. I like those two and I think they will do well together.'

The locals had prophesied this match years ago when Rhuari and Catriona were scarcely out of school. It was often the same on the island. Folk were so familiar with each other that it was easy to predict these unions.

But, despite the inevitability of this match, Mary was excited about the forthcoming nuptials. She was intensely interested in island people and convinced that they were superior in every way to all others, and that Papavray was the only place to live. This opinion was not well based, as the farthest afield that she had ever been was to the busy harbour and fishing port on the mainland. However, Mary's parochial life was never short of interest, as the family affairs and so-called private lives of her neighbours afforded infinite grist to the mill of her incessant chatter.

But she was a good neighbour, always on hand to help anyone, always ready to cook a meal, watch a child, milk a cow, look after an old person or get someone's meat from the travelling butcher. On dark winter evenings, she watched the lane into the village through binoculars to make sure that everyone who worked 'away' got home safely. When it snowed, she knew that Loch Annan would be treacherous and was usually the one to raise the alarm if a villager had failed to appear. Two or three crofters would then set out on tractors, armed with stout ropes, to rescue the latest victim of this notorious hill. A far cry from ringing the RAC on your mobile!

Over the inevitable cuppie, Mary filled in the details about the forthcoming wedding.

'Of course, Rhuari's family is Roman Catholic. I don't think Catriona will change to Roman. Her grandfather was the Free Kirk minister on Rhuna for years, y'see. So I suppose Rhuari will be exterminated . . .'

Startled, I paused with the teapot in mid-air, but then I remembered that this was Mary speaking.

'Excommunicated?' I suggested.

'Aye. He'll have to be or the minister won't marry them,' gabbled this irrepressible lady. 'He's an awful mannie, indeed!'

'But what about Rhuari's mother? Isn't she Roman Catholic? Doesn't she mind?'

'Ach, Peggy's no mindin. She's no been to her kirk for years. Their priest doesna come to Papavray very often, anyway, so he'll likely not know.'

After digesting this surprisingly relaxed attitude to the usually strict Roman Catholic protocol, I asked, 'When is the wedding?'

'Oh, after the lambing and before the steamers, I expect.'

The wedding

It took me a minute to work this out to be April or May. Rhuari worked a croft, so the lambing was important, and Catriona served in a shop near the pier and would be busy in the tourist season, such as it was. But the lambing frequently went on into May, and the steamers began in earnest on the first of June, so I felt that there was a very short 'weather window' here.

Without thinking, I asked, 'Why not after harvest?'

'Too late,' said Mary matter-of-factly. 'The baby's due in October.'

This was something that I hadn't heard about and should have been told in my capacity as midwife.

Rhuari was easily the biggest man on the island and his strength was prodigious, but far from using his Herculean strength to his own advantage he was unfailingly considerate of children, animals and anyone small or frail. Many a cow stuck in the mud or a calf that had fallen into a hollow owed its life to Rhuari. He was well liked and his looks matched his nature, so Catriona would be considered a lucky girl. But she, too, was strikingly beautiful, with blue eyes and dark hair.

'They'll have the dance at the Kilcaird hotel,' continued Mary, still pursuing her current interest. 'It should be a big night.' Island weddings were a great source of excitement and the dance that always followed was a wonderful excuse for a 'big night'.

Mary munched on a shortbread biscuit and then looked at it with a surprised air. 'This is good, Mary-J.' Praise from Caesar, indeed! I was only now beginning to master the art of Scottish cuisine: pancakes, clootie dumpling, Athol brose, proper porridge and so on. The art? Scottish dishes were rather more of a pick-and-shovel sort of cookery!

'Catriona is going to wear her sister's wedding dress. It's a lovely creamy lace, with real court shoes to match.' Mary took a fortifying gulp of tea. 'She'll need to change into the shoes in the porch. Yon kirk path is that muddy under those awful great trees.'

'But, Mary, those are beautiful flowering chestnut trees. They are just coming into bud and by the time of the wedding will be in flower. Super for the photographs.'

'Huh!' Mary snorted.

In common with most crofters, she did not like trees, whereas they were the things that I missed most in the landscape.

'Is Catriona to have any bridesmaids?'

'Aye, of course. Wee Janet and that great lump of a Kirsty from Dalhavaig, I'm hearin. And do you know who is to be best maid? Katy!'

'Katy! Are you sure? Will she be well enough, I wonder?'

'Ach, Catriona will no have her do anything. Just walk up the church and hold her flowers in the service. Katy will be fine.' Mary's faith was obviously greater than mine.

*

Rhuari and Catriona were married on 1 June. The great day dawned bright and clear. Too clear, said the pessimists! The ceremony was at four-thirty, by which time surprised cows would have been milked, startled hens shut up for the night, ewes in lamb left to nature and horses given an early nosebag. The usually grim, bare church had been festooned with flowers, some real and some artificial. The laird's wife had agreed to play the ancient organ, as she was the only person on the island who could coax more than a wheeze out of the tired instrument, which, in this austere denomination, was only used for special occasions.

Amid much coughing and whispering, the congregation assembled. There was a distinct aroma of mothballs. As befitted non-relatives, we sat at the back and so, inadvertently, had the best view of all the arrivals. The hats were amazing! They seemed to range from tight cloches as worn by the flappers of the '20s, through sensible wartime headgear, to 1950s pillboxes, which, when perched precariously on the stiff curls of a fresh perm, bounced alarmingly with every step. The younger women favoured the fashion of the time and were colourful visions in wide-brimmed, much be-feathered creations of every hue. These flapped and fluttered in the draught from the open door so that a group of girls near the back looked like a restless flock of exotic birds.

I turned my attention to the footwear, which was equally diverse. I saw good stout lace-ups, winkle-pickers, patent leather courts, platform soles and fancy buckled affairs circa 1910. It was like watching a pageant. By contrast, the men were boring in their uniformity. Good Harris Tweed suits of a nondescript colour, slightly gaudy ties and brown brogues. At least the wellies had been left at home! Here and there I could see a kilt.

Everyone was impressed by Rhuari. At 6 ft 7 in., Rhuari was resplendent in full regalia: MacDonald tartan kilt, sporran, white socks, skean dhu, black velvet jacket and crisp white jabot. He looked extraordinarily handsome, and his old mother had a proud but startled look as though she could not quite believe that she had actually borne and reared this striking man.

The organ struck an asthmatic note and we all rose

respectfully for the bride. A radiant Catriona appeared in her cream dress with her long, dark, curly hair peeping from below her lacy veil. Her feet were daintily shod in the cream court shoes (changed in the porch, of course).

There was no false sophistication here. Everyone turned to watch and a lot of whispering and nodding went on. Following Catriona was Katy, dainty and beautiful in pale blue. There was an excited buzz as she appeared and, amid the kindly nods and smiles, I noticed that she seemed to have caught the eye of Catriona's brother, Hamish, who was the best man.

The Reverend was oddly nervous, and I couldn't think why because he had conducted every Papavray wedding ceremony for the last 20 or 30 years. I heard the reason later.

Apparently Rhuari had once come upon him rebuking a small boy whom the Reverend suspected of stealing something from the church. He was holding him by the ear and the lad was roaring his protests. The scene offended Rhuari's sense of fair play, so he lifted the holy man bodily and strode to the burn, where he dumped the hapless creature in the water. Since that day, the Rev. McDuff had been ill at ease in Rhuari's presence.

The rain held off just long enough for the photographs to be taken at the church door, and I was amused to see Mary scowling at the chestnut trees.

The evening was a huge success in spite of the thunder that accompanied the band for most of the evening, while the sweating musicians were well fortified with frequent drams at the bridegroom's expense. The old ladies who sat round the edge of the room reminisced about their own weddings of long ago. In their day, weddings were much less formal affairs. The obligatory white dress and smart wear of today was unknown: no one would have considered it necessary to do more than wear one's 'Sunday Best' and make sure that the children had shoes. Life was hard but weddings were a time for fun and dancing, while the ceremony itself was just a necessary part of the day – the excuse for the party. It was still rather like that in the '70s.

Now too old or infirm to dance, the old folk, in their fusty and outdated 'best', tapped their feet and drank their whisky whilst watching the young ones twirling and laughing. Strip the Willow (my boys called it 'Strip the Widow', of course), Eightsome Reels, The Dashing White Sergeant and others were played enthusiastically by the island band. During a brief break for folk to get their breath, Janet played the bagpipes. She was shy but made a lovely picture in her bridesmaid's dress, with the faraway look that she always adopted when playing the pipes. I think she genuinely felt the beauty of the music.

Some of the men spent their time propping up the bar, while two youngsters fell asleep under a table. Fergie, a little the worse for wear, danced with a doormat on his head, and the bride and groom disappeared for a long period of time. There were ribald comments when they reappeared to dance the night away.

My lasting impression of that day was the sight of a radiant Katy dancing with Hamish. Could this be the next wedding?

SIXTEEN

Disaster at Dochart Bay

'Have you no heard the latest?'

Archie was full of the news. He had come over with a rabbit that he had shot, and he and Mary were sitting by the fire drinking a large whisky (Archie) and a cup of tea (Mary).

'No. What?' I was always ready to hear 'the latest' — whatever it may be.

'They are going to build an airport near Dalhavaig!'

'An airport?' George was unable to believe his ears. 'Are you sure?'

'Aye, tis in the *Free Press*. They're beginning next year. It's to be down by the sea near Kirsty's croft, y'mind.'

'On disclaimed land,' added Mary, not to be outdone.

'Ach! The woman means reclaimed land.'

'Hmm,' mused George. 'Any pilot will have to gain height rapidly to avoid Ben Criel.' Avoiding a 2,000 ft mountain within a couple of minutes of take-off would not be easy.

Mary was excited about the project, as yet another of her many cousins was looking for work on Papavray.

'There'll be plenty work while they consecrate the ground!'

We stared at her for a moment. We couldn't think what she meant this time. Then light dawned.

'Do you mean "consolidate" the ground?'

'Oh aye. Something like that.' Unconcerned as ever, she continued, 'They have to stamp it down to stop it from falling into the sea.'

Had this really been the method of runway building, I felt that few people would have much confidence in air travel Papavray-style.

The four of us decided to go and look at the site. We were not alone! Most of the able-bodied population of the island seemed to be gathered at Dochart Bay. Some of the crofters were pacing out various areas with knowledgeable comments.

'It'll no be long enough for this airyplane!'

'They'll end up in the sea. You see if they don't!'

'Well, you'll no get me up in one of yon things!'

Kirsty, whose croft lay nearby, was worried. 'The noise will turn ma cow's milk sour in her udder, it will. Indeed and what about ma sheeps? They'll be droppin lambs like flies, they will.' She shook her tousled head. 'It will no be the same at all!' she prophesied.

It seemed that this wonderful 'airport' was to be a hut, a windsock and a runway, and that was all. The area was at least flat, because it had been reclaimed from the hungry sea years ago for a purpose now forgotten. A tiny lane led to the windswept place and on to Kirsty's croft, and I could see at a glance how dangerously near it was to the lofty heights of Ben Criel. The pilot of a tiny plane tossed about in the turbulent air would have to be skilful, indeed, to take off towards the mountain.

Meanwhile, crofters were telling each other how easy it would be for relatives to visit, children in distant colleges to get home for the holidays and how there would be more 'visitors' to the island. Already, Kirsty was planning to do B&B (in spite of the sour milk, apparently).

Fergie was gazing up at Ben Criel. Suddenly, he said, 'Do you mind that American bomber in the war?'

I was intrigued. 'What happened?'

'It crashed high up on the Dhubaig side of the Ben. Everyone was killed. I was away at sea, but Old Roderick was here.'

We all looked at Old Roderick. 'Aye. Twas a bad do indeed.' He shook his head. 'In bits it was and every single body dead.'

George and I had been children in the war, and we wanted to know more.

Old Roderick perched on a rock under a bank. 'Twas only an exercise,' he told us. 'Getting ready to bomb Germany, they were. Big American plane . . .'

'A Flying Fortress,' prompted Fergie.

'Aye, so it would be,' continued Old Roderick. 'It was at night, rainin and blowin and that dark. No moon – no indeed! Anyways, we were in our beds about two of the mornin, I mind, when we heard the plane. Very low it was – much lower than we had ever known. And then there was this colossal bang! We ran outside and there, high on Ben Criel, was a terrible fire! We could see the flames from the house.'

Appalled, we waited for the old fellow to shift to a flatter rock to continue his story.

'All the men in the village came out and we started to climb up. We had torches and lanterns, and we hoped we might find the crew, or at least some of them, alive, so we just kept going towards the blaze up there. It took us hours and hours!' He paused and appeared to be reliving that arduous climb.

'Well, we started to see bits of the plane long before we got to the crash, but as soon as we saw it, we were pretty certain they would all be dead. Everything was burnt and black. The rain had put the flames out, but most of it was still smokin. Aye, it was a terrible sight, indeed. All those young men in bits. And burnt too! Ten of them, I mind. Poor lads!' He sighed. 'Aye. It was a bad do altogether. There was nothin, just nothin, that we could do. We covered up a couple of them with something or other, but the rest were . . .' He glanced round. 'Aye. Well . . .' He lifted his head and stared out to sea. What were his old eyes seeing?

We were all silent, thinking of the needless suffering and waste of life on Ben Criel all those years ago. After a moment, Old Roderick rose, saying, 'The military came the next day with lorries and ropes and stretchers and I don't know what, and brought the poor chaps down. After the war, some of the American families came over to see where their boys had died. Very sad, it was! They put a stone there with all the names on. It's maybe there still. I've not been up the Ben for years.'

(About a year later, George, Nick and Andy, climbing the boulder-strewn, heather-clad hill, came across this stone with the list of names still visible among the lichen. A sad and lonely reminder of a terrible end to ten young lives.)

Just at that moment, the weather changed. In a twinkling we went from bright sunshine, with the silvery bay reflecting the turquoise of the clear sky, to a fierce wind with horizontal rain beating in from the sea. Black clouds were rearing up from the horizon, and Ben Criel had disappeared altogether. We were now standing on a bleak stretch of wet, muddy, slippery ground. Maybe Mary's 'consecrated' would be a more appropriate future for this place after all!

But long before this 'airport' was built, something happened that seemed so much of a coincidence that one started wondering about 'fate' and the 'paranormal'!

One evening I had picked the boys up from the steamer on their return from a day spent with friends on Eileen Mor. On our way out of Dalhavaig, Andy noticed two large earth-moving vehicles parked as though ready for action at the airport site.

'Can we go and see if they have started yet?' asked Andy.

We were disappointed to find that nothing at all had been done, and we were just turning to walk back to the car when we heard an engine of some sort.

'What's that?' asked Andy, peering round.

Nick was scanning the sky. 'Look! There's a plane – a small one – out over the sea. It looks as though it's in trouble. It's very low! What is it doing?'

The engine noise was all wrong. Nick grabbed my arm.

'It's coming towards us, Mum. It's going to crash! Quick, Andy! Run!'

We ran up the lane, past my car, and crouched behind Kirsty's byre.

The plane came in from the sea, swaying from side to side as it dipped and rose, obviously completely out of control. Then the engine popped, spluttered and died.

With a rush of air, it skimmed the rocks on the shore and with a screeching, grinding noise, the wheels hit the soft sand, bounced and hit again. The nose dipped and the left wing buried itself in the ground. The plane slewed round and crashed into one of the bulldozers. The impact shook the air around us, and the sound of shattering glass and ripping metal was deafening. We watched in horror as the broken body and wings settled into the earth and an eerie stillness replaced the noise.

Nick began to run towards the tangled mess.

'Andy, run up to the main road and stop the first car. Tell them police, ambulance and fire brigade – all three. And get some help!'

Andy set off like a young hare, while Nick and I ran toward the tiny plane, scarcely bigger than the modern microlights. Incredibly, the cockpit seemed to be intact and we could see the pilot slumped forward in his seat. Was he dead? Was he alone? We could not see anyone else.

'Mum, we could get to him by climbing up the wing.'

We scrambled up the slippery wing and reached the gap that had been the cockpit door.

'Nick, go and see if there is anyone else here.'

I eased myself into the cramped and twisted cockpit and looked at the still figure. He was breathing! I felt his pulse. Thin and thready. There was a lot of blood soaking one trouser leg and he had a nasty gash on his head. The seat belt seemed to be pressing too hard on his chest, making his breathing laboured, but I could not reach the clips.

Nick returned. 'There's no one else as far as I can see, but it's an awful mess back there. The tail is hanging off.'

I nodded. 'Come and hold this man up a bit so that he can breathe more easily while I see where all this blood is coming from.'

My surgical scissors were always in my uniform pocket, so I cut away the soaked trouser leg to reveal a gushing wound over an obviously broken bone. 'Nick, apply as much pressure as you can on this bleed.' I pulled a mercifully clean handkerchief out of my coat pocket.

All the time I worked, I had this persistent feeling that there should be another occupant. But the plane was so tiny that

Nick could not have failed to see him. Meanwhile, there was a more pressing problem. Listening to the pilot's breathing, I realised that somehow I was going to have to release that belt. But how? Everything was so bent and twisted that I couldn't get to the catch. I was just about to make use of the scissors again when there was a creak and suddenly the whole plane lurched sideways. Nick shouted, but it was too late! I was flung backwards out of the doorway to slide down the wing and land with a bump on the ground. Regaining my breath (if not my dignity) I looked up and could see that the pilot's seat had been wedged across the doorway and Nick was valiantly trying to maintain the pressure on the wound. I silently thanked the Lord that I had not been able to release the belt or the poor man might have been tossed out after me.

I clambered back inside and between us we stabilised the seat and eventually undid the restraining belt. The pilot's breathing immediately improved, his eyelids flickered and he began to moan. I bandaged the fractured leg to the good one to form a living splint and improvised a sling for what was obviously a broken collarbone. And that was all. We could do no more.

'Oh, what a mess, Nick! I wish someone would come. And where's Andy? I would have thought he'd be back by now.'

'I'll go and see, Mum, if you take over here.'

The bleeding had eased a bit, and I continued the pressure while at the same time trying to restrain the now-restless man. I had nothing to relieve his pain, and all I could do was talk to him and hold him to me for warmth, as it was now getting dark and cold. Time passed while he slipped in and out of consciousness and the plane kept creaking ominously in the gusty wind. I prayed that it would not move again and that help would come, as his pulse was now faster and weaker. I thought of Old Roderick saying, 'There was nothin, just nothin that we could do.' I sympathised.

I was beginning to get light-headed with cold and frustration when at last I saw the lights of several vehicles speeding down the lane. They drew up, and I could see John and Rhuari and the ambulance crew together with the young surgeon from the island hospital. He climbed up and, listening to my comments, quickly examined the pilot, gave him something for the pain and improved upon our makeshift first aid. John and Rhuari stood below, looking up.

'Where are my boys?' I called.

'We are here, Mum,' came two voices. Then Nick said, 'Andy found the other one up the lane. He's in the ambulance.'

At that moment, there was another sickening lurch to one side and the wreckage settled once more. Those on the ground scattered, and the doctor struggled to keep the patient stable.

There was a shout from the fire chief, 'Get out of there! All of you! It's going to turn over.'

'John. Help me,' called the doctor, 'and, Rhuari, get ready to take the patient's weight.' The massive waiting arms of our island giant gently received the patient as he was eased from the twisted wreckage. He was transferred to the ambulance; the doctor leapt in and off it went! John helped me to the ground just as there was a tearing, grinding sound and the whole wreck began to shake.

'Come on!' he yelled.

The body of the aircraft reared into the air, turned right over and with a deafening crash landed again upside down. The doorway through which we had just escaped was now buried beneath several tons of twisted metal. The wing was ripped away and landed bent and jagged among the remains of the bulldozer, and we could now see that the other one was a hundred yards or so away at the tide's edge.

'Bit too close for comfort, that!' said John.

An understatement, I thought. I was beginning to feel that nothing was quite real any more.

Nick and Andy ran towards me. 'What was this about "the other one"?' I asked.

It appeared that on his way back down the lane Andy had come across this dusty figure weaving about in a dazed fashion. He wisely (for a seven year old) made him sit with him beside the road.

The man was concussed with a few bruises but otherwise had had a lucky escape when he had been thrown out of the plane on its impact with the bulldozer. He could so easily have been killed. I heard later that the pilot, Roger, also made a complete recovery.

News of the crash quickly spread, and islanders flocked to the scene to stare at the remains of the first plane to 'land' at the island's airport.

SEVENTEEN

A fragile Fergie and
a shopping spree

One morning I was in the garden when I heard a shout and, looking up, I saw Mary rushing over the croft towards me.

'Mary-J! Mary-J! Fergie's fallen from his ladder.'

I ran inside for my first-aid bag and set off across the village with Mary.

'How bad is he? You might have to come back and phone the doctor for me.'

'He's swearing that bad I canna get him to tell me where it hurts,' said Mary, trying to keep up with my longer strides. Although always scurrying round the village, she was not really built for sprinting over crofts.

We hurried round the corner of the old croft house, whence came some colourful language. There, lying on the coal heap, was a very angry and very black Fergie. This was no time for the normal protocol such as 'reassuring the patient'.

'Did you hit your head on anything, Fergie?'

'No. Just my bloody foot, leg, I don't know! But my bloody wrists hurt like hell.'

'Can you sit up?'

'What? On this bloody coal heap?'

'For the moment, yes. Mary, will you go into the caravan and put the kettle on?'

'I don't want a damn cup of bloody tea!'

'It's not for a cup of tea. We have to wash your face, hands, arms, everything, to see all the cuts and bruises.'

'I could do with a bloody dram!'

I was getting tired of this. 'Fergie,' I said severely, 'will you please stop swearing!'

He looked at me aghast and for the first time seemed to take in who I was and what I was attempting to do for him. 'Oh! Indeed! Oh dear, dear. I'm so sorry! Oh my. I'm so sorry . . . Oh dear, dear!'

'Are you absolutely sure that you didn't hit your head?' These fulsome apologies were almost as worrying as the uninhibited swearing.

'No, no. I know I didn't. This coal arrived this morning. I ordered it a bit prematurely as I have no fireplace yet, but the coal boat was early and I put the ladder on top of the heap to get some extra height. I was going to step onto the roof of the caravan to mend the leak.'

'Can you stand?'

'Aye.'

I helped him into his caravan, where Mary and I washed off the worst of the coal dust. Now I could see that both wrists were swollen and obviously very painful, and his ankle, too, looked angry.

'Can I have that dram now, please?' asked a very subdued Fergie.

'Just a small one. We'll have to get some X-rays.'

Fergie looked alarmed. 'You don't think I've broken anything, do you?'

'I don't think so, but it's possible.'

He groaned. 'I wanted to paint the caravan and start clearing the croft whilst I'm waiting for Callum the Yard to come.'

Callum was a builder from Dalhavaig who had been retained to rebuild Fergie's croft house. We were only too well aware of how long it took to persuade any builder to undertake restoration jobs. They all preferred new-build projects: fewer technical difficulties and more money. Callum had a small business and a builder's yard, hence 'Callum the Yard'. Similarly, we had 'Donny the School' – he was the school caretaker, 'Lachlan by the Shore' – he lived by the shore, 'Rhuari the Pier' – he worked at the pier, 'Roddy the Boat', 'Tormod the Hill', 'Big Craig the Road' and so on. Surnames as well as Christian names were so often duplicated that this method of identification was essential.

The X-rays revealed that he had not broken anything but severely strained and bruised both wrists by landing on them in the coal heap. He had twisted his ankle quite badly too. He was strapped up and decided to go to stay with Mary and Archie for a few days to be looked after and fussed over. Mary would be in her element! Archie, however, put the whole thing in a nutshell, reminding me of Grumpy, one of the Seven Dwarfs: 'Ladders on coal heaps? Bah!'

But Fergie was irrepressible. 'Mary-J, can you add this to your shopping list for tomorrow?' He glanced sideways at Archie and with a wicked grin he added, 'Then I'll not need to put my wee ladder on the coal heap.'

I took the scrawled note from him with suspicion. I couldn't believe my eyes!

'A 30-foot ladder? Fergie!'

An innocent face gazed back at me. 'I'm sure George won't

mind. You have a roof rack on your Land Rover, have you not?'

I gulped, trying to imagine George's reaction.

Our shopping expeditions took place only about three or four times a year, as they involved two sea crossings and one hundred road miles once on the mainland. We had come to the conclusion that these shopping trips were turning into an ongoing nightmare. The fact that we had a long-wheel-based Land Rover had not escaped the notice of crofters and patients alike, and everyone made it their business to find out when we intended to make our next foray into the world of commerce. This wasn't difficult, for I always informed the more elderly or infirm patients of our intentions as they had great difficulty in getting even essentials. But the jungle telegraph swung into rapid action and we were soon inundated with shopping lists. We usually had longer lists for other people than for ourselves! Ordinary groceries and simple household requirements could be obtained in Papavray's small, damp shops, but shoes, clothes, furniture, furnishings, electrical goods, wallpaper, tools and so on all had to be obtained during the infrequent visits to the mainland.

The gentle plea for 'a ball of red wool for the bonnet I'm knitting for Hamish' or the plaintive request for the transportation of 'Annie's teaset that's in the shop but they'll no deliver it' or even 'get Grannie a blue nightie' were taken in our stride. But to these were added such things as a roll of chicken wire, a couple of shovels, a new peat iron, a carpet and so on. Even a big Land Rover had its limits! This time we were also to pick up 'a few little things' from Angus's (another of Mary's cousins) store to bring back for some friends of his.

At 4 a.m., the alarm went off. A quick cup of tea and away!

A fragile Fergie and a shopping spree

It was a spring day and being so far north it was already light when we set off. Nick and Andy were soon asleep again. I revelled in the clear morning air. The sea, for once calm, glistened and the little wavelets were silver in the morning light. The road across the mainland passed between craggy hills already donning their mantle of green and through woods of birch and rowan. Smoke was already rising from cottage chimneys and folk were beginning to let chickens out, rev tractors and drive cows out onto the hill after milking.

We arrived in Inverness at about 8.45. George and I had divided the lists according to our separate areas of expertise. For instance, I would not like to see George buying knitting wool or nighties. As always, we were among the first people waiting on shop doorsteps at 9 a.m., when they opened. Later, we would be the last to be virtually ejected at five-thirty, when they closed.

George was tying Fergie's ladder to the roof rack when I returned to the car with a bucket, a washing-up bowl, a bundle of dishcloths (on offer) and a lavatory brush. None of these purchases was for us.

He was looking very cross and breathing heavily. 'You'd never guess,' he said. 'I rang Angus at his store and he only wants us to take two refrigerators and a dishwasher back with us!'

I stared at him. No wonder he was angry! 'He has sold these, hasn't he, and doesn't want to pay carriage? The wily old bird!'

George's silence spoke volumes. He tied the last rope and off he went. Not a happy man! I was waiting with the boys when he came back with the groaning Land Rover. As we climbed in to set off, we could see a cardboard box wedged between the refrigerators and from it was coming some strange whimpering.

I looked at George. 'Mary's new puppy,' he said grimly.

'And I suppose Mary knew all about this?' I said.

'I suppose so,' said George. He sounded resigned. He shrugged. 'Could be worse, I suppose. Might have been a new cow!'

We got home at 1 a.m. and George gleefully roused Mary to give her the puppy. The rest of the purchases were delivered at intervals between work schedules the next day. Everyone professed to be delighted with the goods and the only thing that we seemed not to have done was complete our own shopping!

The next time we went to Inverness, once again Angus had been told and rang to say would we pick something up for him. He didn't say what it was. When we arrived at his store, we were confronted by a Rayburn! He was quite upset when we refused to subject our backs and our elderly Land Rover to this monster. I was sure that it would have gone straight through the floor.

The gentle pace and intimate atmosphere of the little island shops could not have been more at odds with those on the mainland. Dhubaig boasted one tiny shop measuring about 16 ft by 10 ft. It had one long counter, several wooden shelves, a lot of cardboard boxes and a couple of chairs for the old folk who might have walked two or three miles. The shop was known, rather grandly, as the 'post office', because one could buy stamps, post letters and collect various government pensions there. In addition there was stale bread, jam, canned goods, one or two lines in frozen foods (if the freezer was working) and hen food.

A fragile Fergie and a shopping spree

Old Roderick owned the shop and, although approaching his 80th birthday, had no thoughts of retirement. We happily squelched our way to and fro over muddy crofts and came to accept Old Roderick and his ponderous ways as one of the permanencies of Dhubaig. I was used to having to allow about thirty minutes for a three-minute walk and the purchase of a simple item. Old Roderick spurned pre-packed food, insisting on weighing and packing the customer's required amount of flour, sugar, oatmeal and so on. This was time consuming, but we were content to stand and chat while he plodded to and fro to the old-fashioned scales with a tiny brass shovel. There was an added hazard if one was buying hen food, because he kept that in the byre. He would excuse himself with the utmost courtesy, leave the open cash box fully exposed on the counter and disappear in the direction of the byre. Ten minutes, fifteen minutes would go by and no Old Roderick. On his return there was always a plausible reason for the delay. He would explain with beguiling candidness that as he was in the byre anyway he felt that he might as well let the cows out. Or perhaps his wife had called that she was baking and needed some eggs, so he would potter off to the hen house, and when he took them to the kitchen for her, she might have a cup of tea waiting. He would drain this in a gulp and finally return to his near fossilised customer.

EIGHTEEN

Something on the shore

I was hoeing my weed-choked potato patch one afternoon, when the phone rang.

'Nurse.' It was John, the policeman. 'Can you get to Struakin? I'm there now with a young girl who has fallen from some rocks on the shore.'

'How bad is this and who is it?' By this time, I knew nearly everyone.

'On holiday at Tin Cottage. She's ten. Just bumps and bruises, I think, but there is a biggish gash on her leg and maybe a sprained ankle.' John was used to reporting signs and symptoms to Dr Mac or myself and had become quite an expert on initial diagnosis.

'Did she hit her head?'

There were muttered enquiries at the other end of the crackly line.

'Her mother says not. She saw the fall.'

'Will you stay until I get there, John? It will take me a while, as you know. Keep her quiet. Pressure on the cut if it is bleeding, but you know all this anyway.' He was probably more up to date on basic first aid than I was!

It was only after I had put the phone down that I began to wonder why John was there at all.

Struakin, at the eastern end of the island, was now a village of only four houses. Two of these were holiday homes owned by absentees. The road went only so far and then there was a two-mile tramp over rough ground, but once at the end of the promontory the situation of the hamlet was idyllic. There were the remains of a tiny harbour, a ruined pier and a crumbling sea wall. The houses nestled against the hill and a tiny beach with a sheltered bay made this an ideal spot for a holiday.

It had once been a thriving village with an economy built on fishing, but when the herring shoals gradually failed, first one boat and then another was sold 'away', and the villagers also left to make a living elsewhere. Tin Cottage had once been a corrugated-iron structure that had done duty as the post office, but had been altered to make a small but cosy house, so that the only clue to its humble beginnings was its name. Electricity was absent but oil lamps and open fires had a rustic appeal that drew holiday people to experience a different lifestyle for a week or two. The Johansson family occupied the fourth house. How they supported themselves was the subject of much pleasurable speculation among the island dwellers and some bizarre theories had been put forward.

Packing all that I considered that I would need, I drove to the end of the road and set off on foot to tackle the two-mile walk.

John came out to meet me. 'She's all right, I think. I've had to call in the army . . .' He broke off as he saw my incredulous look. He grinned. 'There's a shell or a bomb or something equally sinister on the beach among the rocks and quite near to the houses. Mr Carter, Caroline's father, saw it when they were carrying Caroline off the shore and back to the cottage.

They rang me to report it, but when I arrived I decided to call you to look at her injuries.'

As we walked towards the cottage, John continued, 'The bomb-disposal unit will probably come in by sea. They might want to evacuate the people here.'

I was ushered into the cottage while John stayed outside to watch for the army unit. Caroline was lying on the settee with cold cloths on her ankle and a white handkerchief tied round her knee. Her facial cuts had been cleaned up and were not serious. In answer to my queries, she said, 'Danny and I were shrimping and Mum was sitting on the rocks, and I slipped and my leg went down between some big boulders. I've lost my shoe!' This seemed to worry her more than her injuries.

She seemed fine, so I just dealt with the knee and we continued with the cold compresses to her ankle, which was swollen and painful. I went outside to talk to John.

'How long do you think they'll be?' I asked, referring to the army unit.

'They should be here any time now.'

'I think I'll stay in case they want to evacuate, in which case I'll strap her ankle to keep it stable. Where will they send us, do you think?'

'Just behind the hills, I imagine.'

'Hmm.' 'Just' behind the hills involved a fair trek over uneven ground. But there were plenty of people to carry the invalid.

We became aware of the throbbing of powerful engines and a rubber boat rather like an inshore lifeboat approached at speed. It slowed and nosed its way through the rocks into shallow water. Two men leaped out and pulled the craft up the beach, while two more busied themselves with mountains of equipment that had been stowed in the bottom of the boat.

The one who seemed to be in charge (captain, perhaps? I didn't notice) obviously knew John, who then took them all off to see this bomb or whatever it was. In no time they were back, looking serious. Giving the device some complicated name, the captain regretted that they could not defuse it but would have to 'effect' a controlled explosion.

'We will need to evacuate the inhabitants to a safe place as a precaution, but there is really no danger.'

Having just heard the word 'explosion', we were not convinced about the 'no danger' bit. I explained that I would have to strap an ankle first and that the owner thereof would need to be carried to the 'safe place'.

Danny, Caroline's eight-year-old brother, was ecstatic at being in the middle of such a drama.

'Cor! Wait till I tell the guys at school!' And to one of the soldiers, 'Hey, Mister, can I 'ave a souvenir after?'

Caroline, too, was excited at being the centre of attention and delighted to be carried to the 'safe place', which turned out to be a hollow behind some rocks on the landward side, away from the blast to come.

We sat in an uncomfortable semi-circle on the damp ground and waited and waited and waited. I'm not sure what I expected, never having been involved in an explosion before (controlled or otherwise), but eventually, when we were tired and hungry, there was a very disappointing 'whoomph' and the patter of some falling debris.

John cautiously poked his head round the rocks. Just at that moment there was a tremendous 'boom' that reverberated around the hills, and John hastily ducked down again. A shower of sand, pebbles and bits of twisted metal could be seen falling to earth some distance away. Nothing touched us in our little hollow. The men had known exactly where to put us for safety.

Two dusty figures came round the rocks and informed us that the device had now 'been exploded' (as if we had not heard!) and we could 'return to our homes'. They must have given these instructions and assurances so many times that they sounded like lines from a film.

As we returned in procession to the houses, Danny was swooping on various bits of twisted metal until his pockets bulged. I thought how envious Nick and Andy would be, and I surreptitiously picked up something that looked vaguely like the pieces of shrapnel that as children we used to collect in the Second World War after an enemy plane had been shot down.

Diarmuid Johansson, his wife and two daughters had been involved in the afternoon's excitement with the rest of us but had said not one word. It was really most odd. One day we were to hear their story.

The men restored Caroline to her couch. Her ankle was looking much less swollen and I thought another day's rest should be all that was necessary.

With good wishes all round, I started the long trek back to my car. At first the path was strewn with bits of rock and rubble from the explosion. Then something caught my eye. There, looking dusty but otherwise undamaged, was Caroline's lost shoe! I took it back to Tin Cottage. Caroline was ecstatic.

When I set off again, the sun was low in the sky and, as I walked, a golden eagle wheeled overhead, swooping to the ground on a high, rounded hilltop nearby.

NINETEEN

Nicholas

Nicholas was growing up quickly. Too quickly, I felt. He still hated Mondays: leaving home at 6 a.m. Monday mornings were 'the pits', according to him.

In all, about 20 scholars from all over Papavray travelled on the steamer to the island of Eileen Mor, where a bus would be waiting to take them across the island to the roll-on-roll-off ferry to the mainland. A school bus met the ferry and trundled off for another 40 or 50 miles to the school itself in the town of Achanach. It was a big, modern affair, serving the senior scholars of many islands and a huge area of mainland. At first, Nick had to stay in the hostel but soon found digs with his friend Basher's grandmother in Achanach.

The old lady was typical of many of the older folk at that time in that she was terrified of nearly all modern gadgets, particularly the 'teleeffission'. One evening, Basher was twiddling knobs, trying to get an acceptable picture, when his grandmother came into the room. She screamed in horror.

'Will ye stop behooterin with the teleeffission! You'll blow us all to Halifax!'

No one could work out why it should be Halifax, but it

illustrated her point, I suppose, as Halifax, Nova Scotia, is certainly a long way to be blown!

At 14 or so, Nick was now a tall lad with a cheery smile and an easy manner. He was also an accomplished mimic and amused everyone with his clowning. He had no trouble at all in attracting girlfriends.

Young people at the school seemed to be very shrewd in their choice of boy- and girlfriend, choosing people from their own island, as they would have had great difficulty meeting in holidays if the love of their life lived elsewhere. The distances, the weather, the steamer or ferry schedules and the cost of travel were all considered. No wonder there was so much inter-marriage on the islands! I remember, however, one notable exception to these self-imposed restrictions.

One of my patients living in Rachadal had a brother who, by the age of 60, had never married. It was generally thought that he was very much under his mother's thumb and certainly he had run her large croft from a very early age.

From her croft, which ran down to the sea, it was easy to see the houses on the shore of Eileen Mor, some four or five miles away over the water. Over there was a similar croft run by a 60-year-old woman for her mother, who was also something of an old harridan, according to local gossip.

How these two met in the first place was never known, but every Saturday, in all but the very worst of weather, old Angus Ben would chug over the water to see Ailsa for the afternoon. He was always back for the milking; he would not have wished to face his mother's wrath had he been late. Ailsa never came to Papavray, but for 30 odd years Angus Ben had made his weekly pilgrimage to court her. Everyone knew that they were only waiting for the two old mothers to die (or 'pass on' or 'pass over' or 'be lifted') and then the 'young ones' would marry.

One summer there was great excitement as Angus's mother did the decent thing at last, so we only had to wait for Ailsa's ailing mother to do the same. And she did, only a couple of months later. The crofters rubbed their hands together: now there would be a good wedding! So everyone waited, and waited, and waited. But nothing happened. Angus was seen crossing the water as usual every Saturday afternoon.

At last, one of the men (I think it was Archie) was instructed to go and see Angus on some pretext to find out how long it was likely to be until the wedding.

After the usual preamble, the question came: 'And when are you thinking of tying the knot then, Angus?'

'Ach, not at all, not at all,' said Angus, to Archie's amazement. 'Y'see, Ailsa has a good croft there and she's of no mind to give it up to her niece. She's no fond of her niece, y'mind.'

'Well, why don't you go and live over there, Angus?'

'What? I couldna do that! Indeed no! I have a good, good croft to me here. What for would I be giving that up to go over there to live?'

So the status quo remained, and Angus continued his chaste Saturday visits to see Ailsa. This went on for many more years until Angus was too old and infirm to make the crossing. They died in their separate beds, in their separate lives, within a week of each other.

In many ways their story goes to show how very wise the young people are to choose partners nearer home. Nick became friendly with Sandy, Basher's sister. Not quite on the same island, but Schula was a bare half-mile off shore. Both families had boats, so it was fairly easy to exchange visits as long as the weather permitted.

Occasionally Nick would go off with George to assist him in some of his work, either on the fishing boats or in small workshops and homes. They often took Pip with them. Pip was a lovable collie but, like Winnie the Pooh, had 'very little brain'. He was very docile, very lovable, very devoted, but very stupid.

One day George was persuaded to wire a house in Cill Donnan. Nick was merely 'the gofer' and fetched and carried all manner of wires and switches during the morning. After a picnic-type lunch, Nick looked round. 'Where is Pip?'

George was busy. 'You go and find him.'

Off went Nick. Since almost every dog on Papavray was a collie, and all collies look much the same, there was no point in asking people if they had seen our runaway. After hunting all through the village, even down to the harbour, Nick was about to give up when he saw the minister get into his car and set off towards the church. Sitting on the back seat, unnoticed by the minister, was a collie dog. Nick knew that Rev. McDuff had no dog and there was something in the benign expression on this one's face as it viewed the passing countryside which convinced Nick that it was Pip. He must have jumped in the car while it was parked outside the manse. The church was several miles away, and Nick felt that the minister was probably going there.

Just at that moment, Chris, a friend from school, cycled into view. Nick hailed him and demanded a lift. Off they went, with Nick's long legs sticking out at either side and his bottom perched on the uncomfortable parcel rack.

'You mind yon daft Callum's gettin wed the day?' shouted Chris to the passing air.

'Oh boy! I hope we'll be there before they start,' bellowed Nick in reply. 'Go faster!'

Every time they went down a hill, the imperfect brakes ensured that they did go faster! Every time they climbed a hill, Nick was instructed to 'get off, ye lazy wee mannie'. In this highly dangerous way they arrived at the church, but not before the bride and her 'maids' entered the door.

They crept round the bushes and peered into the minister's car. No Pip!

Chris said, 'Perhaps he's in the graveyard.'

Nick's search took him past a low window near the front of the building. Peering in, while trying to keep out of sight, he could look at the congregation. They seemed to be a very merry bunch, he thought. The folk in the front pews appeared to be making much use of hankies, not to dry the usual sentimental tears but to cover their red convulsed faces. They were all trying desperately not to laugh!

Nick froze as an awful conviction assailed him. This had something to do with Pip. He was sure of it! He edged round a bit and the minister came into view. There seemed to be nothing amiss there, except that his Reverence was looking rather puzzled as he led his merry congregation in the solemn marriage service. Nick's gaze roamed around until he happened to glance at the window on the opposite side of the church and a little behind the minister. There, in the slanting sunshine on the wide windowsill, was Pip, basking in the warmth!

The people could see him, but the minister could not – as yet. The dog only had to yawn loudly and Heaven itself would be hard pushed to save him from a booting by the holy man, for he was not a dog lover. Dogs were not God's creatures, according to him. Apparently, the devil had put them on the earth.

Chris had joined Nick and together they held a whispered conversation.

'Can we get in the back way?' asked Nick.

Chris knew the kirk well. 'Yes. There's the vestry door.'

Together, they crept into the vestry. The door into the body of the church was ajar and they could hear the monotonous voice announce a hymn. Hymns were only a concession at weddings, as the Reverend did not approve of them.

The boys heard the old organ take an asthmatic breath and launch into 'Love Divine'. As soon as the voices of the congregation reached a crescendo, Nick gave a short whistle. Pip lifted his head and looked towards the vestry door. The singing became a little wobbly as the singers watched the drama. Nick held his breath as Pip rose from his perch, stretched and jumped down to the floor. The minister, intent on leading his people in their devotions, noticed nothing. Not so the congregation. Nor the bride and groom!

'Come on, Pip! For heaven's sake, COME!' rasped Nick, somewhere between a shout and a whisper.

Ever obliging, the dog strolled across behind the black-robed figure (no white robes here, even for a wedding) and started towards Nick. Then he thought of something that he needed to do and with a beatific expression walked back to the ground-hugging robes and cocked his leg. The stream of urine soaked the austere garment and, having made himself comfortable, Pip ambled to Nick, wagging his tail in greeting. This was just too much for the wedding guests, and the hymn singing broke down entirely as uninhibited laughter took its place. The good Reverend finally became aware of something unusual and even the organ groaned wheezily to a stop.

Before the wrath of God, or at least His representative, could catch him, Nick grabbed Pip and all three raced out of the vestry door, through the churchyard to the gate, where they had left the bike. The two boys leapt on and Nick shouted to the dog, 'Come on, you stupid mutt! Ride, Chris, as fast as you can, until we're round the bend!'

Once out of sight of whatever retribution might be following them, they collapsed onto the grass and hooted with laughter.

'Oh, man!' gasped Chris. 'Yon preacher's wet through!'

'Did he see us?' wondered Nick.

'I don't know, but Callum and Mairie did. And all the rest.' Chris could scarcely get his breath for laughter. 'Yon will be a good tale at the weddin feast.'

'But the minister will be there!'

'Ach, no. He'll no be there at all,' Chris reassured Nick. 'He'll be on Eileen Mor. Callum got his aunt to ask him to go over to give her the Communion after, because he didna want the old misery at the weddin breakfast.'

'Not so daft after all, then,' said Nick.

TWENTY

God's country

Every spring, we began to dig peat, plant potatoes and generally gear up for the busy months of summer. So by May, everyone was getting ready for the 'season' in one way or another and hoping for good weather for the 'visitors'. But some folk came back to our 'sceptred isle' every year no matter what the weather threw at them. These folk loved the peace and the open spaces, the uncluttered roads and the unsophisticated lifestyle. They toured or walked, fished or climbed, or perhaps just leaned on a bar and chatted with the locals, or maybe sat on the harbour wall and watched boats coming in and out. They enjoyed all the simple things and welcomed a holiday that recharged them for another year.

On the other hand, there were some who couldn't stand the quietness and roamed around in a disgruntled fashion looking for 'nightlife', grumbled about the steep hills and lack of buses, and proclaimed to the world that they were bored. These people never returned.

During the summer season, Dr Mac and I became used to treating all manner of minor ailments. We even had cases of sunburn, because the heat of the summer sun in the islands (when it deigns to appear at all) is always underestimated by the visitors. There is usually a cooling breeze to fool the unwary, and the air is so clear that every ray reaches the skin of a sun worshipper. So clear, in fact, that aircraft, flying so high that they appear as mere dots on the roof of the world, will throw their shadows to the ground, where they seem to creep along among the heather on the shaggy hills like some weird moorland creature.

One glorious day in spring I was 'in the peats' at our peat hag high on the hill near Loch Annan. We had cut the brown wet rectangles in April, throwing them onto the tussocky grass to dry. The weather had been kinder than usual, so they were now hard and light, dry and crumbly. When the peats reach that stage, they have to be stacked in pyramids of about 50 or so.

I was taking a rest, sitting on a bank, gazing at the quiet loveliness of the view, listening to the merry song of skylarks and watching a distant eagle scooping up the sky with its huge wings. It soared high in the blue dome while it scanned the ground for an unwary mouse or cheeky fox cub. The peace was complete, encompassing my world and seeping into my very soul.

A slight rustle made me turn to see someone skirting the far peat bogs. As the figure drew nearer, I became intrigued. Here, out on this lonely hillside, walking at quite a spanking pace, was a priest in full garb! The black soutane flapped in the cooling breeze and the figure clutched a beretta in his hand. It occurred to me that he was probably as surprised to see a woman sitting in a peat bog as I was to see a priest in clerical clothes walking the hills.

He drew near. 'What a wonderful day! It is good to be alive on such a day.' A man after my own heart! We exchanged pleasantries and introduced ourselves. Father Peter MacAnally was from Southern Ireland, with a delightful accent to match. He was young, handsome and very tall, the soutane streamlining him even further. Looking at him, I could see how young women might fall for this forbidden fruit, and I wondered if he found this difficult.

Gesturing a request, he seated himself beside me and gazed out over the hills and the sea to the far mountains. A sigh escaped him.

'This is wonderful! This is what I came for. I'm walking on several islands for charity. This is truly God's country!' He grinned rather sheepishly. 'The charity bit is wearing this ridiculous outfit in order to be sponsored.'

'What charity is that?' I asked.

'A local one for a small girl who was badly burned in a bomb attack on the border. She is going to need complete care for the rest of her life, and her parents have very little to offer being rather . . . um . . . mentally challenged, is the term, I believe.' He sighed again. 'I work in a very poor area of Dublin. All this is just fantastic.' He made a wide sweep with his arm.

The distant black and purple mountains were so clear that the dark corries and jagged peaks seemed only a mile or two away. The crystal sea sparkled with moving golden light while the deep valleys below us drowsed in the blessed warmth of a crimson spring day.

I said, 'It is all so clean and pure that it looks as though God finished making it all today and He has only just gone.'

Father Peter smiled and said, 'Oh, no. He hasn't gone. He is still here, all around us.'

I looked at my watch. The school car would soon be bringing Andy and another young scholar back from school to their homes in Dhubaig. Andrew would be 'starving' as usual. I invited Father Peter home for some refreshment, and we made our way towards my car on the distant brown ribbon of road. The peat hags were mercifully fairly dry or the ankle-hugging soutane would have become sodden with dark peaty mud. What a ridiculous requirement for sponsorship!

Father Peter and I climbed into my little car and set off across the high open moors that lean on the side of Ben Criel. This narrow lane beside the peat bogs was inclined to sink under the weight of moving vehicles and rise again after they had passed: it virtually floated on the boggy ground. We were used to it, but strangers to the island found it difficult to believe that the road would not sink altogether.

We had come to the point on the narrow road where it plunged downwards. Below us glittered the dark waters of Loch Annan, which contrived to look menacing even in brilliant sunshine. As we began the descent, I saw Father Peter clasp his hands tightly together, whether from dread or in prayer I could only guess.

'Papavray!' he said suddenly. 'A strange name, is it not?'

'Well, not really,' I replied. 'I think it means "priest isle", so you should feel quite at home. "Papa" is an old Norse word for "priest", I'm told. I don't know how it strayed to the Hebrides; it is more suited to the Shetlands or even the Faeroes. But there is a legend about a hermit who came here in early Christian times and converted everyone.'

We reached Dhubaig and descended the track that led to our croft house. Father Peter paused in the 'garden' to admire the view of mountain and sea. 'Garden' was a polite term for our 'small acre' of grass, a few bushes and some bedraggled potato plants. But the garden was still beautiful, with its burn bubbling through the wilderness and meandering its watery way to a tiny stony cascade before leaving our land to wander off towards the waiting sea.

A mackerel sky was developing, indicating the end of a beautiful afternoon. Before dark, the rain, borne on the wind, would fall with myriad sharp, painful, flint-like drops. We knew our capricious weather only too well.

Once inside, Father Peter tucked into clootie dumpling, which he appeared to enjoy enormously. Even George had been forced to admit that my dumpling now rivalled the expert baking of my more experienced neighbours.

Andrew came running across the croft from the school car, rushing to avoid the threatening storm. He exploded into the house, propelled by the bullying wind. His cheery greeting fizzled to a halt when he saw Father Peter sitting beside the fire. Even in the summer, we needed a fire in the evenings.

A little in awe of the black-robed figure, Andy recounted his day in a subdued tone and then startled me by saying, 'There's a new girl in my class.'

I had not heard of any recent arrivals on the island, and I already knew all the 14 or 15 island juniors as a result of my monthly health visits to the school.

'Her name is Fiona. She's English.' The succinct information came in disjointed outbursts between mouthfuls of dumpling.

Andy continued, 'Her mum and dad have taken Tin Cottage for a year.'

Another surprise, as Tin Cottage was usually only let to holidaymakers.

'Her Dad's a nature . . . um . . . nature . . . ist?'

Father Peter's eyebrows nearly disappeared into his hair.

Hastily I said, 'Naturalist, perhaps?'

'Well, flowers and bees and things. She's a bit funny,' Andy went on, munching happily.

'How do you mean "funny"?'

'Well, in the head, you know.' And with that, we had to be content.

The storm was increasing: we could feel the buffeting of the wind on the stout walls and hear the thunderous sea crashing on the shore. The room was almost dark by 6 p.m., as restless Stygian clouds streamed across the sky.

George was away on one of the many east-coast fishing boats, testing the sonar equipment. This necessitated a short trip to sea.

Hesitantly, I asked Father Peter what his arrangements were for the night. To ask him to stay was out of the question with George away. I could just imagine the interest that would cause!

'Oh,' he said offhandedly, 'I have a tent near Coiravaig. I was on my way back to it over the hills when I saw you.'

I stared in disbelief. 'A tent! In this?'

'Oh, it's quite substantial. I'm not supposed to stay in inns or B&Bs. The sponsors would be most unhappy. I think they rather like the idea of their priest having to "slum it" in a tent. You see, I usually have a housekeeper to look after me.'

With a sigh, I settled for driving him the two miles to Coiravaig, taking a thermos of tea and some food. The tent was sturdy enough and had been pitched in a relatively sheltered spot, but . . . After inviting him for lunch the next day, I turned the car and drove home, thankful for the bright warm home with the crackling fire and pungent smell of peat smoke. It poured and blew all night, and in my wakeful moments I wondered how Father Peter was coping in that little tent.

God's country

Next morning dawned bright and brittle, pretending that it could do no wrong. But we knew that this sunny splendour would not last, for we could already see more rain clouds hiding behind the mountains. Although it was late spring, the pasture was still sparse, so one of my morning chores was to take hay to Sunshine, our Highland pony. We had bought her soon after our arrival on Papavray when we found how very inexpensive it was to rent a vast field near Dhubaig. Although no expert, I had always loved riding and I was keen for the boys to enjoy it too, but they seemed to prefer fishing. So Sunshine was not ridden as often as she should have been and frequently became naughty and difficult to control. But by this time, we all loved her and were resigned to her cantankerous ways. She was reluctant to embark on an outing and needed much encouragement to leave her field but always galloped back to it as soon as we turned for home. There was a bridge nearby made of wooden planks. Sunshine did not care for this bridge at all and preferred to avoid it altogether by plunging into the fast-flowing burn that ran beneath it, soaking the unfortunate rider. And yet she would ostentatiously avoid walking in puddles. I had decided some time ago that I had a lot to learn about ponies.

I approached the concrete shed near the house. Stored within it was chicken feed, dog food, cat food, saddles, harnesses, multitudes of tools and Sunshine's hay. I opened the door.

There, curled up on the hay, wrapped in an old horse blanket, was Father Peter! The tent had blown away during the night.

TWENTY-ONE

Farewell to Chreileh

It was an exceptionally bright and calm day as I made my way to the surgery one morning in May. The grass was a vivid green as young shoots pushed their way through the cold soil; the thin bleating of new lambs could be heard and ewes gratefully gobbled their fill after the privations of winter.

Dr Mac was bustling about as I entered, which was most unusual. He was normally a man of measured step, serene countenance and calm speech.

'Nurse, I have to get through surgery quickly this morning and you must do just the essentials with equal speed. We are to go to Chreileh.'

At the mention of that small remote island, my heart lurched and the terrible memory of Biddy and her plight came flooding back. Chrissie, who often came to Papavray to visit her sister, had kept me informed of all the preparations for the evacuation of the island, but, as with every venture involving the Hebridean seas, they had to wait for a calm day to get the old people, the remaining livestock, the furniture and the crofting equipment off the exposed and inhospitable isle in a succession of small boats. It seemed that today was the day.

Dr Mac was telling me that we were needed to supervise the removal of the two infirm old ladies.

'I'm told that Mrs Macintyre might need sedation; so far she has refused to be moved,' he said.

'Where are they all going?' I asked.

'Well, Angus and Chrissie and Donald and Dolleena will get cottages here on Papavray, near the castle, because the men are to work on the estate. The two old ladies will need care and assessment in the hospital and then they'll go to the home on Rhuna. There is no one left to look after them now, as both families are abroad. The rest of the men are off to the mainland for work. It's all very sad, but it has been inevitable ever since the whaling stopped and the fishing declined.' He sighed. 'The end of a way of life.'

The depopulation of the Hebridean islands began at the time of the notorious Highland Clearances, continued through two world wars and still went on today, as employment was easier to find on the mainland. When yet another family left, the crofters would say, 'Ach, there's one less light in the village.'

Here and there, however, there was a glimmer of hope as someone's grandchildren took over a croft, or another family arrived to start a pottery or B&B or a shop. One of the ruined castles on Papavray was to be stabilised to house a rural-life museum. The building of the long-awaited airstrip and the resurgence of interest in the Gaelic language all helped to bring employment. We watched and hoped that the tentative regeneration would gain momentum. Looking back now, I realise that we were witnessing the beginning of a new and hopeful era, much of it based on tourism. Most of the Hebridean islands are now enjoying a degree of prosperity undreamed of when we first knew Papavray.

Farewell to Chreileh

Dr Mac and I boarded one of the locally based fishing boats in Dalhavaig harbour for the long trip to Chreileh. Nearly 20 men and a large number of women were coming with us in a small flotilla of boats. It would take muscle and time to move all the paraphernalia of the lives of several families.

The pale sea sparkled in the sunshine and little white horses romped quietly in the gentle salty breeze. Contrasting with the turquoise sky, the grey and white wheeling seagulls were resting on the docile updraught. Oystercatchers, with their unique cry, were skimming the water, undeterred by all the activity. An Atlantic seal popped his head above the waves to see what all the commotion was about; with his bright, intelligent eyes and cheeky whiskers, he reminded me of a wet Labrador dog.

What a contrast this was to the conditions the last time we came to this rocky isle. I raised my face thankfully to the warm sun, but in spite of the beauty of the day and a certain thrill at being part of this drama I was sad, for I could imagine how the crofters would pine for this remote rock when it was left abandoned in the vastness of the North Atlantic.

At last we neared Chreileh. It contrived to look uninviting even in the sunshine, with its ruined croft houses and derelict sheds. The narrow channel to the old pier meant that the larger boats were forced to stand off until full tide, while the smaller clinker-built boats, manned mainly by crofters, came alongside.

I could see that the whole operation was going to be complicated and difficult, especially as I had spied two large Shire horses! What was the story behind the presence on the island of these two, I wondered? Croft work was invariably done by the sturdy Highland ponies, and it was the first time that I had seen Shires in the Hebrides.

A small knot of people was standing on the pier surrounded by boxes, bundles, crude crates of squawking chickens and various pieces of furniture. Several collies were circling a small flock of sheep; two men were approaching, driving four cows and three very young calves. As the first boats approached the pier, there was a loud babble in both Gaelic and English as everyone voiced their own opinion as to how things should be done.

'I'll have half the sheeps in my boat, but Angus will need to take the rest,' declared Johno, a bearded giant of a man.

The captain of one of the bigger boats was eyeing the Shires. 'I'll need to be taking those two, I'm thinkin. But how am I to get them onto the boat? Why did you not think to tell us about them, Douggy?'

'Ach, I forgot.'

'Forgot?' The enraged captain blew his cheeks out. 'How can anyone forget a coupla tons of horse?'

Things were not going well!

At the other end of the pier, the women were loading the smaller pieces of furniture and personal belongings onto Archie's boat.

'Enough, enough! Tis no the *Queen Mary*! I'll be takin some of this lot out to Tammy's boat. Then I'll be back for more – if I don't sink on the way.' Laughing heartily at his own joke, Archie pulled on the rope and started his engine.

'We'll need to get Wally's boat alongside. Tis the only hope for the horses.' A worried-looking Douggy seemed, at last, to take in the difficulties. So long as a boat could get alongside the pier, some wide, sturdy planks (very sturdy planks) could be put in place (like a gangplank) and the calm, sure-footed beasts could be led onto the deck. But the larger vessels had deeper draughts and could not get in at the moment. The only hope was when the tide was full.

Dr Mac was watching the proceedings. 'I think we'll go and see our patients. I can't imagine that things will move smoothly.'

Chrissie met us in the low doorway of an old so-called 'black house'. 'Mrs Macintyre is in here. She's been hollering that bad I canna do anything with her, Doctor.'

We followed her into the dark, low-ceilinged room and had to wait for our eyes to accommodate to the gloom after the bright sunlight outside. In spite of the warm weather, and the imminent move, a peat fire burned in the crude fireplace and an incredibly old lady sat beside it. She was dressed in the style of some 60 years ago and, to my utter amazement, she was smoking a pipe!

'*Ciamar a tha*!' came the usual greeting.

'*Tha gu math*!' we replied, but as that was just about the extent of my Gaelic I left Dr Mac to do the talking while I persuaded the old lady to allow me to remove the pipe and peel off the many layers of clothing so that the doctor could examine her. All the time, she ranted loudly (presumably about the move) and Dr Mac answered quietly.

He straightened up. 'She's as sound as a bell. No problem at all. Just old age, I think.'

He turned to Chrissie. 'How old is she?'

'We were thinkin it must be a hundred and one or two. No one knows exactly, but we were tryin would we work it out the other day. She remembers things happening way back in 1872 and believes that she was about three or thereabouts. She had her son in 1886 at around fifteen, so . . .'

'No birth certificate?' I asked.

Chrissie shook her head. 'Not many of the old folk have.'

As I dressed Mrs Macintyre, she became quiet. I think she was beginning to realise the futility of her objections in the face of the inevitable. She was frowning and then huge silent tears fell down the wrinkled cheeks. Suddenly, the ranting harridan turned into a frail old lady, grieving for her home and the way of life that she was about to leave for ever. What had the poor soul to look forward to? Wrenched from her home, her neighbours, everything she had ever known, she was to be borne off to another island, which, to her, might as well have been another planet.

We moved on to the next croft house, accompanied by the compassionate Chrissie, who seemed to be the self-styled carer of both old ladies. Here, we met Mrs Cameron: a very different kind of person. She was quiet and frail, blind and completely bedridden. This lady spoke English, and I was surprised to hear an unmistakable English accent. She had come to Chreileh 60-odd years ago to marry a young seaman she had met in a mainland town. He had been killed before their only son had been born, but she had stayed on among the kindly folk of the island. Her son was now in Canada and she rarely saw him. Now this! And yet here we had a gentle, uncomplaining lady, prepared to cooperate with everything that was envisaged for her. I was deeply affected by her story and her courage.

She was talking to Dr Mac. 'Well, you see, Doctor, it's not so bad for me because I am not a native. The island does not mean as much to me: none of my ancestors lived or are buried here.'

'But you have lived here for 60 years and raised your son here. I would say that you are just as much a Chreileh woman as any other.'

'No, Doctor. It's not the same. Everyone has been good to me, but I'm still an incomer, you see.'

An incomer still after 60 years? What hope was there for us, the MacLeod family, on Papavray?

Dr Mac pronounced both ladies fit to travel. Some of the men would carry them to the boat when it was time to leave, so we retraced our steps to the pier.

The place was a hive of activity. Small boats laden with boxes and bundles and bits of furniture were chugging to and from the bigger boats, which were standing off. Once there, ropes were lowered and precariously held objects could be seen rising to the decks. As usual, everyone had his own idea how to do things and proclaimed it loud and long.

The patient Shires were still on the quayside, quietly chomping in their nosebags, but, as we watched, Wally's boat gradually inched its way towards us, slowly negotiating the narrow channel.

Roddy came to stand beside us. ''Tis worth a try now the tide's in, but t'will be turnin in a wee whiley. Then it will be worse than ever. T'will dry out entirely! If he makes it, they will have to move the beasts gie quick.'

Everyone watched as, inch by painful inch, Wally brought his craft nearer. The crowd was now quiet, holding its collective breath. Closer and closer came the boat at a maddeningly slow pace. But Walter could not afford to create a bow wave, as that would cause more mud to slither into the already shallow water. After what seemed an eternity, there was a scraping of steel on stone as the old craft reached the pier. There was an audible sigh of relief from the watchers and then a terrific babble broke out.

'Hurry you now. I'll have the Shires, but I canna risk the

weight of the sheeps as well. You'll be needin to take them to Malcolm's.'

'But we'll have to hoist them up from Archie's boat!'

Archie looked aghast for a moment. Then he began to chuckle. 'Well, they do say that pigs might fly, so how about the sheeps? But John will need to take some or the tide will beat us.'

The huge Shires were gently led aboard Walter's boat and were as cooperative as ever, as though they were quite used to this maritime experience. The captain kept a worried eye over the side as the horses' great weight was added to the already laden boat, but at last the placid animals were on the deck and he began to go astern, even more slowly than he had approached. Once more we watched with concern (and a degree of awe) at the quiet confidence of this experienced man.

Meanwhile the 'sheeps' were being urged aboard the smaller boats by the busy collies. Two or three at a time were the most that could be safely carried in a tiny craft to Malcolm's boat, so Archie and John had to make many trips. Once alongside, slings of sacking attached to the ropes that had been used for the furniture were lowered and placed around the sheeps' bellies. Large hands held the woolly beasts from below, passing them to those above, whose strong arms received the terrified animals.

Walter was steaming away towards Papavray by now, with the Shires' majestic heads raised to the wind. Hitched only loosely to the superstructure, they were still unperturbed. How I love and admire these big, brave, placid fellows!

Dr Mac was getting worried about evening surgery. He approached Chrissie.

'Do you think the men could fetch the ladies now? I want to travel with them and time is getting on.'

Chrissie departed towards Mrs Macintyre's house, calling to someone as she went. A little while later I could see one of the tall young men who had been helping at the pier effortlessly carrying Mrs Macintyre, who was swathed in coats and shawls in spite of the warm day. Chrissie followed with blankets, a pillow and an ancient suitcase.

Once aboard, I busied myself making the old lady comfortable in the little cabin while Chrissie and the young man went back for Mrs Cameron.

'Here we are then.' They entered the tiny cabin with the second burden. Mrs Cameron was as quiet and compliant as ever and thanked everyone for helping her. The young man discreetly withdrew.

'I'll help you to settle them,' said Chrissie. She looked at me sideways with a little smile on her face. 'Do you not know who that is?' she asked.

Busy with my patient, I said, 'No. I haven't seen him before.'

'No one had until today. That's Johnny!'

I looked at her uncomprehendingly.

'Our Johnny! Biddy's Johnny! My nephew.'

'Chrissie! How wonderful! Tell me all about him.'

But I had to wait, for at that moment the shout went up. We were off!

The pier, such a hive of activity for so many hours, was now deserted. Dr Mac and I watched from the boats with the rest, as a silence fell on the previously vociferous crowd. It was a sad feeling of finality, for this was an island that would never be inhabited again. Everyone watched as Chreileh, their home for so many years, faded into the gentle mist and was left to mourn its lost identity.

Or perhaps not? For humankind is transitory, while the

mighty cliffs and the raging sea will go on for ever. In the millions of years since Chreileh's creation, and for the millions to come, *Homo sapiens*' brief presence here is only a moment in the existence of this lonely rock that men have called 'Chreileh'.

TWENTY-TWO

The return to roots

A dark shape slipped silently into harbour and the man brought his tiny craft alongside, among the fishing boats. The night was dark and stormy with scudding clouds and lashing rain. No one saw him.

The crews of the bigger boats were either asleep in their cottages beside the harbour or in their bunks on board, oblivious of everything – even the roaring wind and crashing seas.

The man climbed the slippery stone steps, carrying the bow and stern ropes and secured them to iron rings set into the wall of the quay. Head down against the weather, he returned to his boat. Scrabbling about in the tiny forward cabin, grumbling the while, he picked up a large and rather lumpy grip bag, made sure that the zip was adjusted to his liking and ascended to the quayside once more.

With his torch in one hand and the bulky bag in the other, he battled his way through wind and rain to the steep little town. Part way up the hill, some tiny squeaks began to come from the bag.

'Ach. Haud your wheesht, you!' growled the man. 'Aye. The sooner I get rid of you, the better.'

The town was in darkness, but he could see some lights at the top of a hill.

'Ah! That will be it,' he muttered.

'It' was the little cottage hospital. There was a stout front door with an old-fashioned bell beside it, so, transferring the bag to the other hand and turning his torch off, the man pulled on the bell. The discordant jangling grated on the quiet street, and he glanced nervously around. The noises from the bag were now more insistent, and he stamped his feet impatiently. He felt in his pocket for an envelope, which he then stuffed just inside the zip. At last he heard footsteps approaching and bolts were drawn back. Light, spilling from the door as it opened, seemed to punch a hole in the darkness and rain.

A sturdy young nurse peered out and, taking in the scowling face and rough appearance of the man, was about to shut the door when she heard the whimpering coming from the bag in his hand.

Suspicious, she asked, 'What do you want? And what's in that bag?'

Without answering, the man stretched out his arm and pushed the bag towards her.

Turning, he strode off into the night.

The nurse had automatically taken the bag from him, fearing that he would drop it if she hesitated. By now she was worried by the increasing noise coming from the contents. An animal? Puppy? Cat? Or . . . ?

She sat on a nearby chair and, pulling the bag onto her lap she began to unzip it. She gasped as she peeped inside. There, wrapped in a grubby blanket, lay a very tiny baby!

'Sister! Sister Bailey! Come here. Quickly!'

The return to roots

A well-starched and fairly substantial lady came into the hallway.

'What is all the noise about? Patients are trying to sleep, Nurse Mackenzie, and you . . .' She broke off as she became aware of the crying baby in the old bag and looked at the white, shocked face of the young nurse.

'May the Good Lord save us!' she exclaimed. 'And what wickedness do we have here?'

She bustled forward and gently took the screaming little bundle out of the bag. Cradling the child against her bosom, she began to soothe and rock it. She looked enquiringly at the nurse.

'A man rang the bell. He handed me the bag. He ran off . . . I . . .' The poor girl was too shocked to continue.

'Who was he?'

'I didn't have time to ask. He ran away so fast and it's dark and . . . Oh! What are we going to do? Is the baby all right?'

'First things first,' said Sister. 'The child is cold and probably hungry,' she sniffed. 'And most definitely dirty,' she added.

'Nurse, make up a bottle of milk from the maternity ward and bring a napkin and a clean shawl. We will wash and attend to the child in my office, as it is warm in there. I'll undress him or her to see if the little soul is all right or if there has been abuse,' she added darkly.

She hurried off, carrying the now-quiet little bundle. In the office, she removed the blanket (tutting at the dirt) and then the clothes. She was surprised to see that the vest and nightdress were clean and well made. The napkin, although soiled, was of good soft fabric and carefully pinned. Gradually, a little baby boy emerged, quite well nourished but cold. There were no bruises or other marks on him, and he appeared to have been well cared for.

'I do not understand,' muttered Sister Bailey. 'You are beautiful, and I think you have been loved. But how did you end up here, in a dirty grip bag, in the middle of the night?'

All the time, she was crooning comfortingly to the child as she wrapped him in a cot blanket.

Nurse Mackenzie came in with the milk. Sister Bailey offered the bottle to the child, who sucked with vigour and contentment, snuggling into the starched bosom with little snuffly noises. She washed and dressed him in the newborn-size garments that the hospital stocked, and he finally fell asleep in her arms.

'Right,' she said, becoming her usual efficient self. 'What do we know about him? Anything at all? Bring that filthy bag in here and we will see if there are any clues as to his identity.'

Nurse Mackenzie placed the bag on the floor and pulled another blanket out. Then she noticed something.

'There is a letter. Look!'

Sister Bailey motioned her to open and read it. The nurse pulled out a single sheet of lined paper, obviously torn from a notebook of some sort.

It said: 'Bastard child Johnny 1 month Free Kirk.' Nothing more.

This bald, unfeeling statement was all that the man (whoever he was) had bothered to tell them.

'Oh, the monster!' Sister Bailey looked at the sleeping baby. 'Well,' she said. 'At least we know your name now. Hello, Johnny.'

She addressed Nurse Mackenzie. 'You saw him. Do you think he might have been the father? How old do you think he was?'

'A bit too old to be the baby's father, I would have thought.

Fiftyish, perhaps. I don't know. He was very rough-looking and sort of brutal. He didn't seem to care at all. Just couldn't get away fast enough.'

At that very moment, the man was speeding away through the choppy sea as fast as his old boat would take him. He was scowling and muttering to himself.

'The wickedness of the flesh! Keep her out of sight. The woman, too, but she'll not last long.'

The wild, mad look was replaced by a sly and cruel grin.

'No one will know. Tell them she's gone away? Aye, we'll tell them she's gone away.'

Chuckling unpleasantly to himself, he chugged his erratic way out to sea and was soon swallowed up in the darkness.

In the light and warmth of Sister's office, Baby Johnny slept in the encircling arms. Looking at the sleeping child, she sighed and murmured almost to herself, 'How could anyone not want this adorable child?'

Then, resuming her usual businesslike air, she said to the nurse, 'In the morning, we will tell Matron. The police will have to be informed and we will get Dr Donald to check baby over. Then, I suppose, he will go to the children's home while they try to trace his parents.'

'I wish we could keep him here a while,' said Nurse Mackenzie. 'Just until we know what is to happen to him. Perhaps Dr Donald might want to keep him under observation,' she added hopefully.

Sister shook her head. 'You had better get on with your work.'

Johnny slept until 6 a.m., when he was changed, fed, cuddled and settled down again. Matron was informed in the morning. As the baby's story spread around the building, he had many doting visitors. The doctor considered that he was remarkably well, considering his journey through wind and rain in an old bag.

'How long was he travelling?' he asked. No one knew.

'I shall inform the police and we can hand him over to the Sisters at the convent. They will care for him until he is identified.'

'Doctor,' interrupted Matron. 'I am told that he comes from a Free Kirk background.' She showed him the note.

'Ahh,' said the doctor, rather at a loss. He stroked his chin ruminatively. 'Trouble is, the nearest Free Kirk children's home is away down in Glasgow. We don't want the wee chap to have another long journey at this stage, do we? It will have to be the Sisters for now.'

'The Sisters', or more properly 'The Sisters of the Convent of the Holy Sepulchre', were only a few minutes' walk away. Wondering if she was doing something religiously reprehensible, the Matron contacted them.

Mother Superior did not seem worried at all. 'Indeed, Matron, would the Good Lord be mindin who looked after His children? We will baptise the blessed soul immediately. It would seem unlikely that he has received this sacrament already.'

The Mother Superior prattled on. She was very Irish and very garrulous, but everyone knew how kind she and the Sisters were. So Johnny was carefully carried down the street and placed in their care.

And so began another chapter in the short but already eventful life of Baby Johnny.

Sister Theresa, a young novice, was given the care of the baby. Coming from a large Irish family and being the oldest girl, she was very experienced and capable. Mother Superior, with wisdom and compassion, had realised that Sister Theresa was not suited to the life of a nun. She was just waiting for the right moment to suggest that she left the convent.

'Am I thankful to the Good Lord that I hadn't told her,' thought Mother Superior and departed to the chapel to convey these thanks to the Higher Authority.

Meanwhile, far-reaching enquiries were being made by the police and children's authorities. The sparse information about the man, the clothes and the letter was followed up and led nowhere; adverts were put in various publications and all the Scottish newspapers. Nothing.

Johnny grew into a sturdy toddler, deeply attached to Sister Theresa but at ease with all the nuns, who were enchanted by him. Mother Superior worried that it was an unnatural environment for a child, so when he approached school age it was decided to have him fostered with a family well known to the convent and situated nearby. This way he would have the company of other children and a more natural home life.

Mr and Mrs Mackay, unable to have a family of their own, had fostered countless children over the years. When Johnny joined them, they had one other child, a little girl called Geraldine, who had, like Johnny, been abandoned. Her mother had been traced to a prison in England.

So the children grew together, played together and went to the local school together. They were about the same age, but as no one knew the date of Johnny's birth, he was given the same birthday as Geraldine, so that there could be a big joint celebration each year.

Both children knew that they were fostered but not the details in either case. They were so happy with the Mackays, whom they called 'Gran and Gramps', that the occasional remark that they overheard seemed not to worry them at all. Through the years, the police occasionally came up with some 'lead', as they called it, but Johnny's parents were as elusive as ever.

When the children reached the age of 16 and were both at the grammar school, Mother Superior, now very old but as wise as ever, felt that they should be told the true circumstances of their birth, in so far as they were known, and subsequent abandonment.

Both children listened to the gentle voices telling them such strange and diverse stories. Geraldine was asked if she wished to see her mother, but she was adamant that Gran and Gramps were her family and she wanted nothing to do with the woman who had abandoned her. Johnny found it difficult to believe that absolutely nothing was known of his family or place of origin. He too was happy with Gran and Gramps, but with a boy's natural curiosity he wanted to know more. Mother Superior promised to ask the police to renew their efforts to find something, anything, that might shed light on the darkness of his beginnings.

Gran and Gramps would talk about the way that Johnny was developing.

'He's a good boy,' Gran would assert. 'But he should be doing more school work.'

'Ach, leave the boy be,' Gramps would answer. 'He must have been from farming stock, I'm thinking. He is a natural with animals. Maybe he'll go into the farming when he leaves us.'

'Ach, wheesht, you!' Gran hated to think of the day when both her charges would be leaving to make their way in 'the big wide world'.

'We have him for a whiley yet. He might go to college. Perhaps he'll be a vet.'

But far away, on a small, wind-bruised island, a discovery was being made that would change the course of Johnny's life.

Biddy had been found!

Suddenly, everyone knew that a baby had been born to Biddy about 16 years ago. Sadly, she could tell the authorities nothing, as her inhumane treatment had injured her mind beyond hope, but right from the beginning the local police had been involved in the terrible drama as it unfolded on Chreileh, so the connection was soon made.

Gran, Gramps, Mother Superior and various officials gathered to break the news to an unsuspecting Johnny. A multitude of emotions roared through his mind and body as he learnt of the death of his father and heard the tale of his mother's long years of imprisonment by her half-brothers in the farmhouse. He heard of her eventual release and her present whereabouts in the nursing home.

But his mother had loved him! It was obvious from the diary of her mother that Biddy had loved him deeply for the short time that he had been with her. This was of paramount importance to him.

Johnny remained in shock for several days. He gradually adjusted to all that he had been told and even found himself assuring Gran and Gramps that they were still, and always would be, his family.

So Johnny was taken to visit his mother. She did not know who he was at all: she only smiled and nodded. But he could see that she was sweet-natured and he readily believed that she had loved him. He realised that he could not even imagine the pain she must have felt when her baby was so brutally taken from her. Through his tears, he promised to visit her again soon. Then he set off for Chreileh – the isle of his birth and where, he had been told, he had an aunt who was waiting for him.

He was only just in time. On the very day of Johnny's arrival, this lonely isle, which had seen his birth and all the pain and wickedness that had surrounded it, was abandoned for ever.

TWENTY-THREE
Andrew

BEING A YOUNG CHILD WHEN we went to Papavray, Andy was luckier than the other three, spending the best years of his childhood in the freedom of the island. Elizabeth and John enjoyed visiting, but the island could never really be home, as they had their own lives elsewhere. Nick had some good memories of his time there, but at 12 onwards boys are beginning to leave childhood behind, so he had missed the best years in which to be a part of such a wild, free environment.

I suppose it was inevitable that Andy's best friend was Thomas the factor's son, the only other stranger to the Gaelic tongue, and the two spent much time together and often stayed overnight in each other's homes. Thomas was three years older than Andy and was therefore the leader in most of their exploits. The factor's house was near a rocky bay not far from Dalhavaig, and Thomas and Andy spent many happy hours there with fairly primitive fishing rods. I don't remember ever being asked to cook any fish, but they had fun!

One day in early spring, Big Craig was trudging along the road from Dalhavaig to Cill Donnan when he heard shouts and yells from the direction of the shore. At first he could see no one, but he turned off the road and down through the bushes towards the sea. Emerging from the cover, he looked down on the waters of the little bay with its multitude of tiny rocky islets. There, on the largest and farthest away, were two bedraggled figures surrounded by the swirling waters of the incoming tide! They were yelling their heads off in an attempt to call attention to their plight. Being so intent on their fishing, they had failed to notice that they had become marooned on their rock and that the smaller ones towards the shore had disappeared beneath the sucking water, leaving none of the footholds over which they had jumped so joyfully a few hours previously. Now they were terrified!

Big Craig shouted to the pair, 'Stay where you are! You're no to try to get back. The current's too strong. I'll be with you on yon rock in no time!'

Sturdy though he was, the waves and the suction of the swirling sea around the rocks buffeted him from side to side. Soon the water was above his wellies, so off they came. They floated away and then sank in the open sea. Soon he was up to his thighs and still he was not at the rock.

'Take off your boots!' he ordered. The water was now lapping at their ankles. Big Craig battled on, flinching as the sharp stones and shells on the seabed bit into his bare feet. He noticed the boys trying to hold on to their boots and fishing gear.

'Leave all that,' he shouted. 'I canna take all yon!'

He arrived at the rock at last and, extending his massive arms, told the boys to catch hold of his hands.

'You'll be gie wet but no matter.'

They were reluctant to enter the cold spring sea, but a sharp tug from the big man unbalanced them and they landed in the choppy water in two splashy belly-flops. Big Craig was now up to his waist, but, holding each boy's arm in his huge hands, he forged his way towards the shore, dragging them horizontally across the water.

Two more crofters had now arrived on the shore and they helped the cold, wet, exhausted trio onto the pebbles. Andy and Thomas coughed up a great deal of seawater and were then very sick. Big Craig just sat on a rock staring out to sea.

'I'll no see ma boots again,' he muttered. He seemed totally unaware that he had just saved the lives of two very foolish little boys!

Someone had called the island ambulance, which was based at Rachadal hospital a mere half-mile distant. Checked over in the hospital, rubbed down and wrapped in blankets with their feet in the smallest white theatre boots that could be found, the boys were no worse for their watery brush with eternity. Big Craig was also cocooned in a large blanket, but his feet were so big that nothing could be found for him to wear, so he sat barefoot waiting with the boys for Richard and George to fetch them. (I was on duty elsewhere and only heard about all this on my return.)

Next day, the two miscreants and their parents arrived at Big Craig's house. He was obviously amazed to receive more than the perfunctory thanks of the day before. He refused money for wellies but accepted the offer of a lift to the crofters' store, which was the only place where he was sure to get some big enough. The boys had brought him chocolates (most locals were virtually addicted to chocolate) and were sincere but subdued in their thanks. I think they had both had the worst scare of their young lives. Just before we left, Richard said, 'A bit deeper and you'd have had to swim for it, Craig.'

'Ach. Not at all!' said Big Craig. 'Not at all! I canna swim. I never learnt!

To this day, Andy bears the scars of his next flirtation with doom.

*

Sometimes, during school holidays and weekends, Andy went with George to the fishing boats or to Papavray boat yard. He enjoyed this and felt equal to the island boys, who often worked with their fathers on the croft or at the fishing.

One Saturday morning, I had just driven home after a very light morning's work and was planning a relaxed afternoon. As I opened the door, the phone was ringing. Unsuspectingly, I dumped my bag and hat and lifted the receiver.

'Mary-J! Andy has been hurt . . .' It was George.

I sat down on the stairs with a bump.

'He's been hit by a block and tackle, and the doctor is here now. You had better come.'

'How bad is he? Tell me how he is. Is it his head or what?'

'Yes. But he has come round now. He'll be all right. Just come and get him.'

And with that I had to be content. Come round? So he had been unconscious! And what was a block and tackle?

Heart thumping, I raced back to the car. I was up and over Loch Annan as fast as the rutted road allowed, all the time wondering what damage, temporary or permanent (horrors!), Andy had sustained.

When I entered the boat yard and saw the pathetic, white-faced, blood-stained little figure, I was horrified. Andy was sitting on an old chair in a little hut that was obviously used for making tea. When he saw me, he burst into tears. George was standing by the door.

'Where's Dr Mac?' I wanted to know.

Andrew

'He's had to go. Someone has fallen off a cliff somewhere. When I told him you were coming, he said to take him to Rachadal hospital for stitching – if he needs it.'

'Have you been sick?' I asked Andy.

'Yes – very! And my head hurts.'

I looked at the gash on his forehead. Luckily he had been hit on the front of his head rather than the back. (A bang on the front is less likely to cause as much damage.) But there was so much blood, in his hair, on his face, clothes, even his shoes, and the whole place was so unsanitary that I thought the best thing to do was to bundle him into my car and make for the hospital without delay.

'What was it that hit him?'

George went to the hut door and pointed. 'The block and tackle.'

A huge square steel or iron affair hung from the roof and attached to the underneath was an enormous hook.

'It's used to haul engines out of boats and lift other heavy stuff. It was the hook that hit him,' said George.

The staff was ready for us and the efficiency of this small but excellent hospital swung into action. Andy was X-rayed, assessed, cleaned up and three stitches were inserted. We could now see that his pupils were normal size and equal, and he said that his headache was not as bad. His colour was beginning to return, and he was no longer tearful. He had been very lucky indeed!

He did not know it, and I doubt that he does to this day, but I spent the night on the floor, beside his bed, unconvinced that he had got away with such minor injuries when I thought of the size of that hook.

TWENTY-FOUR

Wedding bells (without the bells)

At about Easter time, excitement began to be felt in the MacLeod household. Elizabeth and Paul, home from college, were busy making plans for their wedding, which would take place in the summer. Lists of guests were flourished about, and when George saw the length of them his face took on a haunted look. The families on both sides were fairly extensive, and hordes of college friends were also to be invited.

The local Church of Scotland minister, the Reverend McDuff, was contacted and the exact date fixed, then the hotel for the reception and dance, then the band, cars, flowers, clothes and myriad other things considered. All this would be stressful even in the south, but there were many difficulties to be overcome on a small, remote island.

An appointment was made for the couple to see the minister almost immediately, as they would be back at college until close to the date of the nuptials.

On the evening of the interview, Paul and Elizabeth made their way to the manse. The door was opened by the minister's stern and weatherbeaten sister, who told them that 'Himself' was in the garage and would be in shortly, and would they care for a cup of tea while they waited? Declining, they sat stiffly in the cold, damp study for some time. Finally, the door opened, but it was Miss McDuff again to say that they had better go round to the garage themselves, because 'Himself' appeared to have forgotten and she had to go out to a meeting.

They obediently went round to the back of the manse to seek the elusive and forgetful minister. At first the garage appeared to be empty, but then a figure emerged from beneath an elderly Morris Minor.

'Ach. It's yourselves! Indeed, I had forgotten. I'm having a little trouble with the manifold but I think I have fixed it. The Lord be praised!'

For a moment, Paul and Beth were not quite sure if the praise, thus offered to the Lord, was for the car's manifold or whether they were supposed to bow their heads in prayer. But the good Reverend began wiping his hands on an oily-looking rag in a very businesslike manner and peered short-sightedly at them.

'You'll be the nurse's daughter,' he averred. Then, looking severely at Paul, he continued, 'And you are to be joined to her in holy matrimony.'

Both nodded and turned to go back to the cold study, but to their surprise the minister sat himself down on a handy oil drum and indicated that they were to sit on a rather grubby bench nearby. He began his (obviously much-used) pep talk. There seemed to be a great deal about the evils of fornication and very little about the joys of married life. Perhaps this was because he was a 60-year-old bachelor! He thundered on about the sanctity of the married state but kept glancing at the Morris, obviously more interested in returning to his beloved car than instructing the two young people in the importance of the step they were about to take. The actual wedding arrangements were only briefly touched on, as the holy man seemed to think that the usual service would be followed verbatim. He was most surprised when the two young people expressed a few ideas of their own but grudgingly agreed to these modest changes. However, when Beth mentioned 'bells', the poor man nearly had apoplexy!

'Bells? Bells? Those heathen sounds? Oh no, no, indeed no! We have no bells in my church, and we certainly would not ring them even supposing we had. Dear, dear!'

Finally he rose, obviously feeling that the two were chastened, shook hands with Paul, calling him 'Hamish', ignored Beth almost entirely and was on his way under the car before they had left the garage. The two arrived home in a dazed state, wondering if the Reverend would remember to emerge from his garage to marry them at all.

They went back to college for their last term. Telephone calls flew back and forth. A few weeks later an enormous box arrived bearing the legend 'Bond Street Bridal Wear'. When George saw it, the haunted look deepened.

I was very busy, as the arrangements for an island wedding are very much a do-it-yourself affair. The cars were a disappointment. Beth had set her heart on a white Rolls-Royce. Unsurprisingly, there was not one on the island so the local garage (the only garage) produced a white Mercedes. Where this came from, we never knew.

The hire of a band was another problem. The island group was remarkably proficient in Scottish dance music and Celtic ballads but knew nothing of 'that English stuff'. In the event, it didn't matter, as the youngsters thought it a great laugh and happily leaped about to reels and Gay Gordons. Well, they were in Scotland, after all!

The biggest problem, I thought, was going to be the accommodation of some 30 people, all of whom would have travelled 600 or 700 miles by land and sea. Students are not known for their wealth, so I could not just expect them to go to the B&Bs or the hotel, and our house would be bursting at the seams with Paul's parents, Beth, her bridesmaid and the four of us.

I need not have worried! As soon as the jungle telegraph got going, the offers of 'a wee room for the two nights' were pouring in. In no time at all, beds had been arranged for all the guests. I was amazed and grateful to so many generous people.

The summer term ended and Elizabeth arrived with an enormous number of bags and cases. The following day was spent on the phone, assuring nervous motorists from the south that, although they were primitive, we did have roads.

I had insisted that the kindly hosts should not have to feed the hungry hordes as well as house them, so it was arranged that everyone would come to our home for meals. As eight was the maximum number that our table would seat, this meant three sittings of eight people, three times a day for two or three days, depending on the length of time that each was staying. Quite an undertaking!

At last, the great day arrived. The weather was fine, the kilts swung and the top hats remained where they should, as there was no wind. The ladies' dresses were beautiful, but they all had trouble with their high heels on the uneven ground. Elizabeth was a vision in *the* dress and even George appeared to have lost the haunted look. The Scottish service was undoubtedly strange to most guests, the organ was its usual asthmatic self, and we all knew about the bells! But none of this seemed important as Elizabeth and Paul, looking proud and happy, were joined in holy matrimony.

The minister disappeared quickly after the blessing. I expect he preferred to be under his car. I'm sure he felt that we were all beyond redemption anyway.

The photographs were taken in glorious sunshine on the lawns of the hotel, with a magnificent backdrop of mountains and sea. When the midges began to join in the photo session, everyone trooped inside to eat a hearty meal.

I began to relax for the first time in weeks. My cup overflowed when the Scottish dancing (much of it on the lawns) was a huge success, and I felt that I could congratulate myself that there was nothing left to go amiss.

I was wrong.

The guests had all gathered outside the hotel to wave the happy couple off on their honeymoon when one of the 'well-oiled' crofters staggered and fell backwards against the very substantial wall of the old building. His head made loud and sickening contact with the granite, and he fell to the ground unconscious.

The usual flurry of activity followed, and the evening ended with the departure of the island ambulance, bearing the now-vociferous crofter, who was claiming that it was all due to the sherry that we had 'made' him drink, having nothing at all to do with the many whiskies he had purchased at the bar during the dancing.

I collected him, personally, from the hospital several days later. He was still blaming the sherry!

TWENTY-FIVE

Searching the seas

'Oh, Nurse, I can't make out what's botherin her. I can't at all. She's never wanted anything to do with the little soul from the day that she was born,' Ina sighed. 'But now, suddenly, she's wantin to know how much feed she has and how do I make it up, and how often do I change her and what does everything cost.'

'Isn't that a good thing, Ina, that she is taking an interest at last?'

'Aye, but y'see, Nurse, she still doesna want to hold or cuddle the wee child. It's all too quick. And another thing, the headteacher wrote that she's been skippin school, and the hostel says that she's often late comin in in the evening.'

Jaynie was at the same school as Nick, on the mainland, so she had to stay in the hostel from Monday to Friday.

'Perhaps she is under some pressure. Or maybe being teased about the baby. Perhaps even ostracised by some of the children. Would you like me to have a word with her, Ina?'

'Aye. Perhaps that might be best. She'll no listen to me at all.'

Ina was caring for Jaynie's baby, as I had known she would. At thirteen (fourteen now), Jaynie was certainly not ready to be a mother to her four-month-old baby, but to ignore her altogether was odd. Fourteen-year-old girls usually get quite 'gooey' over babies. So Jaynie's complete rejection of her child seemed to point to some deep-seated problem, but now she was suddenly showing an interest? I had an uneasy feeling about this.

'Ina, what has happened to Callum-Ally?'

'Ach, he's in another home on the mainland. I hope they keep a good eye on him. Angus says he's very resentful and sometimes they have to sedate him because he gets violent. Oh, Nurse! I wonder what I did wrong that I gave birth to a boy like him. A boy? Huh, he's near 30 year old now.'

There were tears in her eyes and a lifetime of suffering on her face as she shook her head, blaming herself for Callum, for Jaynie, for the baby.

'Ina. None of this – none of it – is your fault. You have been one of the best mothers to your own children and to baby Janet. You have nothing to blame yourself for. I will have a word with Jaynie. Does she know now that Callum-Ally is her brother?'

'Well, we told her, but she didna believe us. Just thought we were makin it up so that she wouldn't see him again. Now, she won't even talk about it at all – just walks out if we try. Dr Mac is goin to tell her what is wrong with Callum, try to make her understand. As for baby, I'm just thankful to the Good Lord that she seems to be normal so far.'

'And is Callum still a secret from the island as a whole? None of the family has said anything?'

'I think it is. Oh, I hope so. I do indeed! I couldna deal with it all, foreby, if t'were to come out.'

The following day, I tried to have a productive talk with

Jaynie, but my hopefully gentle questions were met with grunts, and when I mentioned 'Callum' she turned and walked away. As I left, I noticed her picking the baby up from her pram and holding her awkwardly at arm's length, looking at her and then putting her down again. When she saw me, her face took on a defiant look.

Early next morning, the phone rang.

'Nurse, Nurse! She's gone! She's taken the baby! Angus is away for John. What will I do? What will she do to the wee soul?'

A storm of weeping followed in Ina's frantic call.

'Gently, Ina. I'll call Doctor. Do you have any idea where she has gone?'

'No, Nurse. She was just gone when I got up. What can have happened? She has no money to speak of, so where will she go? Some of her things and the baby's stuff has gone, and some baby food but not enough for long. I'm not knowin if she will look after wee Janet all right. And it's cold . . .'

'Any relatives or friends that she might go to?'

'Angus is away to see. I've tried everyone near us, and Douggy and Benny [Ina's sons] are lookin too. I'm goin to the post office to be near the phone for the police and so on. I don't know what else to do.'

'That is a good idea, Ina. You can see your house from the post office in case she comes back.'

'Nurse, she doesna love that wee child. Will she harm her? Will she?'

'The first thing is to find them, Ina, so I'm off to help.'

I looked out of the window. There was a grey blanket of fog hovering over the sea, which meant that the air would be cold and damp. How much clothing had that silly girl taken for the baby? Had she learnt enough to care for her? This must have been planned – that is why she had been asking Ina all those questions.

Telling the boys to search our side of the island and spread the news, I drove to Dalhavaig post office. Ina saw me coming.

'John's just been,' she burst out. 'Rhuari and Daft Arnie said a young lass with a baby was picked up by a man in a boat at the harbour back a few hours ago. Someone's got them! Someone's taken them! What will I do?'

Overcoming my alarm, I said, 'Ina, from what you said about Jaynie having taken clothes and so on, it looks as though she has gone willingly, doesn't it?'

'But who is this man that they saw?' Then her sobs stopped and a look of comprehension came over her face. 'Oh, dear Lord, it's Callum-Ally! They've let him out again. The fools. The fools! Or he's escaped. He is not fit for anything, Nurse. And a boat!' She was nearing hysteria.

These were my own thoughts. Jaynie must have been seeing him near the school. Whose idea was this and where were they going in a small boat in choppy seas with a tiny baby? I tried to comfort Ina, but what hope could I give her? At that moment, Angus appeared.

'Angus,' shouted Ina. 'It will be Callum-Ally in the boat. Ring the home.'

'I have. Callum failed to return from an afternoon's supervised walk yesterday. Some supervision! And they didn't think to tell us. We could have been on the watch, the stupid . . .'

Angus's jaw moved as he strove to keep calm. He was very angry, but as a devout Free Kirk Elder he was trying to contain himself. He took Ina into his arms – an unusual public gesture for an island man.

'He must have been very persuasive and she is undoubtedly in denial, either about his identity or his mental state – perhaps both,' he murmured. 'God help me, but I wish they would lock him up for life. I'm cold with fear for them.'

I, too, had been remembering that Callum was often violent now.

'Have they any idea where they might be headed?' I asked Angus.

'Rhuari said they turned out to the west. He shouted after them. He was tryin to warn them about the sea and the weather. They took no notice, just turned out to sea.'

Ina rocked to and fro in torment. 'They'll all be drowned out there, they will.'

'Hush, you,' instructed Angus. 'Rhuari raised the alarm and now everyone knows tis an emergency. They have launched the life boat from the mainland.'

'But that will take for ever!' Ina would not be comforted.

Angus coughed. 'They have Roddy's old boat. It's no too fast a boat . . .'

'And no too safe, foreby,' added Ina. 'So they have stolen a boat as well. Oh the dear Lord! Thieving now!'

'What type of boat is it?' I asked.

'Outboard, 14 foot, small forward cabin.' Rhuari had joined us. 'There will be a bit shelter in the cabin.'

'So long as the fog holds off, they should find them soon – unless they hide among the rocks . . .'

Angus left the sentence unfinished, for we all knew that to hide among the jagged rocks was no better a scenario than remaining out to sea.

He continued, 'The coastguard vessel is nearby and will be searching, and several of the men have launched their boats too.'

'What do we do now?' Ina was near to collapse.

I spoke up. 'You stay at home, Ina. Morag and Mary-Anne will be here in a minute to keep you company. You could put a hot water bottle in the baby's bed and make sure there is plenty of baby milk in the house. Heat plenty of water and see there are warm dry clothes ready.' This would give her something to do, although I felt that a hospital bed was a more likely destination for both when they were brought in. If they were brought in. They had not even been sighted yet.

I had to complete my patient round and then I went to Dr Mac's house. News would come via his phone or John's. The doctor's house was near the harbour, so we would be nearby when (if?) they were found and brought in by boat.

Dr Mac, Fiona and I sat and waited. So many people were out hunting that there was little we could do at the moment, but we might be needed later. From the window I could see more small boats being launched and fanning out to the west. There were two tiny islands to the west: Ardnacloich was inhabited and Lachach Isle had been uninhabited for the last hundred years or so. Could they be making for Lachach Isle? There were some ruins still on that isle.

I mentioned this to the doctor, who seemed to think it a possibility and rang John, who contacted the lifeboat, which set off in that direction.

We jumped as the phone rang. Dr Mac listened while Fiona and I held our breath. His shoulders drooped.

'No sight of them. But the lifeboat is not anywhere near Lachach Isle as yet. The fog is getting worse, especially on the mainland, so there is no hope of the helicopter joining the search. Some dozen or so private boats are out, mainly searching the Papavray coast. Who knows what that stupid pair might do?' He thumped the arm of the chair he sat in. He was very angry. 'What is the girl thinking? Surely she could see that a baby ought not to be subjected to a small boat in the open sea. That girl needs psychiatric help as much as her brother!'

I had never heard Dr Mac raise his voice in anger. It was obvious that he was very concerned for the lives of Jaynie and the baby. I had a sudden worrying thought of my own.

'Can I use your phone, please?'

I rang home. I brought Nick and Andy up to date with all that was happening and then fiercely forbade them to put to sea in our small boat to help, as I had feared that they might.

'I want you to go round the headlands near Dhubaig and Coiravaig and look in all the bays that you can see. And alert Basher. He might see . . .'

'I have already, Mum. He and his parents are searching their coast and waters.'

Doctor, Fiona and I waited again. Fiona made some tea and we waited some more. There was no moon. Did they have a light? Had they taken enough baby milk powder? Did they have clean water to mix it? Warm water? And what was the weather doing now?

As though reading my thoughts, Dr Mac turned the ancient wireless on for the weather forecast. To our horror, gales were forecast for the Hebrides. The phone rang, but it was only an update from the coastguard HQ.

'No real news yet. They might have landed on the north shore of Papavray. Their boat is incapable of much speed, so they cannot have gone beyond the area already searched. Apart from the lifeboat and the coastguard, there are about 20 boats of various sizes out looking. But is just possible that they are on

Lachach Isle, and a search party has just been put ashore there.'

'I feel useless here,' I said. 'Now that the search has been extended to these shores, I think I could be of more use over in our area, which I know so well.'

And with that I drove home, changed into warm things and joined the dozens who were already scouring the shores, rocky outcrops and bays on the north side of Papavray.

From the headlands, we could see the powerful beams of the coastguard vessel as it swept the surface of the sea, picking out the tops of the waves and turning the white spray into golden showers. The 'thrum' of the lifeboat engines was loud as it nosed its way in and out of the dangerous rocks near Papavray and the islands of Lachach and Ardnacloich.

Suddenly, we heard the sound of a foghorn. Once, twice, three blasts! This was not the normal, doleful sound of the usual strictly timed warnings.

'They've found something – that's what that means,' shouted Archie. 'Come on!'

Back over Ben Criel we went with Nick, Andy, Rory and Big Craig all packed into my car. We were excited but already dreading what the boats had found. Were they alive? Were they safe? Uninjured? The baby?

As we approached the harbour at Dalhavaig, we could see the lifeboat ploughing through the tumult of the sea in the deteriorating weather, slowing to negotiate the notoriously difficult entrance. We leapt from the car and ran to the quay. We strained our eyes to peer through the gloom, trying to see onto the deck. Then one of the crew on board raised his hand in our direction with his thumb firmly in the air. They were safe!

Ina and Angus rushed up the gangplank, and Dr Mac and I

followed them into the cabin area. There sat Jaynie, wet and bedraggled, with blood on her face and hands, crying uncontrollably and clasping the baby. Wee Janet was very pale, wet and quiet. Too quiet! Ina rushed to Jaynie and took the baby in her arms with scarcely a glance at her daughter. She took one look at the tiny soul and turned to me. I was unzipping my warm padded coat and ripping open the two cardigans beneath it. I took the baby, Ina held on to the wet blanket, and I clasped the child to my body, wrapping the cardigans around us both while Ina, quickly understanding, zipped up my coat. This is the best way to warm a baby in an emergency – body heat. It would do for now.

The ambulance was on the quay. Dr Mac and Ina jumped in, while a grim-faced Angus carried Jaynie. I was helped in with my little burden. This baby was cold and floppy, pale and far too quiet. Her eyes were open, but they had no expression in them. She was in a very bad state.

The staff of the little hospital was ready, and the patients, parents and Dr Mac disappeared into its warmth.

I went slowly back to my car. My involvement would be later, when Jaynie and little Janet came home. If Janet survived, I reminded myself unhappily. She was in a critical condition.

I was just drawing away when I spotted John. 'Where is Callum-Ally? I didn't see him in the lifeboat,' I called.

John shook his head. 'No. The coastguard took him to keep him away from the other two. He didn't seem to be hurt, but he'll be assessed on the mainland and then probably locked up. He is obviously quite deranged.' John rubbed his head. 'What on earth possessed that place to let him out? And what was young Jaynie thinking of, to risk her baby like that? Och! It's beyond me.'

'I think she needs treatment too, John. We failed to realise that the trauma of the birth had had such an effect on her. She seemed all right, and Ina was so good with her and the baby that we were too confident. But Callum-Ally must have been extremely devious and persuasive to get Jaynie to agree to such a stupid and dangerous undertaking. Where were they found, John?'

'On Lachach Isle. The lifeboat chappies found them. They were in one of the old ruins. No roof, no floor, no fire – nothing! Just huddled in a corner. Jaynie seemed relieved to be found, the chaps said, but Callum-Ally tried to fight them off, shouting that they were to get off "his island". He seemed to think he owned the house and the whole island, daft devil that he is! They should lock him up and throw the key away!' And having delivered himself of this uncharacteristically venomous opinion, John marched off.

I realised that John probably knew of the brother/sister connection. Not that it mattered now – it would never be a secret again. Callum-Ally would have to be dealt with, and it would undoubtedly be in all the papers. But that was all in the future. It was the present that was important.

Jaynie recovered physically, but she was withdrawn and uncommunicative, and still ignored her baby altogether. Little Janet hovered close to death during the first few hours: she was seriously hypothermic. Ina never left her side, and after a day or two she was out of danger. Sores caused by clothes soaked in salty seawater took days to heal, and the state of her little bottom showed that her napkin had not been changed at all. She needed a lot of persuading to take her bottle, frequently vomiting the contents. I think her stomach had been affected by the cold milk that Jaynie had given her during that terrible day. As I had feared, they had not taken any means of heating milk or water.

But gradually she recovered and was taken home to be loved and cherished by a relieved and thankful Ina. I visited every day for some weeks, and my respect for that family knew no bounds. Not only had they to deal with the delicate baby and Jaynie's withdrawn state and Callum-Ally's criminal acts, but the publicity as well. The newspapers had a field day. But Angus and Ina were stoic. Their faith upheld them, they said.

There was still a long, long way to go for this family before they could know any real peace of mind: I felt that this was still only 'the end of the beginning'.

TWENTY-SIX

Shearing in the sunshine

I climbed the hill ahead of everyone else so that for a short while I would have the solitary peace that I so enjoyed. I was on my way to the sheep fank, high on the heather-clad hills that rose steeply behind Dhubaig. Soon, eight or ten crofters would arrive together with their wives and their collie dogs. We were going to shear the sheep!

The woolly beasts, belonging to all the crofts in the village, would be gathered by the busy collies and herded into the fank – a stone pen.

Today, it was the turn of the ewes with lambs at heel. They were always sheared later in the summer than those who, for some reason, had not produced a lamb. Those who had were allowed to keep their wool while the lambs were still young and needed to snuggle up to their mothers' warm flanks during the chilly nights.

In an hour or so, the hillside would swarm with people, and the clamour of whistles and shouts would pierce the quietness. Laughter, too, would ring out over the glen, to bounce back from the far hills. The islanders always found something to laugh about in the most unlikely circumstances – stress, exhaustion, sadness even. But for now I sat amid the quietness of this flawless day.

Nothing intruded on my solitude except for the sound of the distant sea, where gentle waves erupted shoreward and fronds of seaweed ululated in the shallows. A cheeky robin perched on a nearby bank and watched me with his beady little eye. Maybe he knew that the presence of humans meant an abundance of crumbs. But the most evocative of all the wild wilderness sounds was the call of the curlew. There is a legend which claims that the call of the curlew aids the spirits of the dying to leave the body and travel to the next world. This idea might have been of great comfort to the folk of old.

I enjoyed these days, when I could work alongside the crofters, watching and understanding their practical skills, their ingenuity and their cheerful acceptance of the hardships of life. To the rest of the UK, crofting may seem archaic, but in times of real hardship – drought, flood, earthquake, and so on – the crofters would be likely to survive far better than those with more 'up-to-date' lifestyles. They reared their own animals, grew their own crops; they dug peat for fuel; they had always been frugal with water and other resources. They knew the moods of the sea, could read the weather and so on: all the skills necessary for survival in cataclysmic circumstances.

But my ruminations were interrupted as, gradually, this all-encompassing serenity fractured and I became aware of the voices of the men, the twitter of women's chatter and an excited bark or two as the crowd puffed its way up to the fank.

'Ahh. It's yourself then, Nurse! You are gie early, foreby,' Morag called as she heaved a heavy basket of food onto the wall. She sat thankfully, breathing hard. It was a very steep hill.

Archie, Mary, Fergie and Old Roderick, who was at least 80, arrived next, carrying various bits of rope, bags of animal feed – in case bribery proved necessary – and some cans of water for the dogs, as there was no stream nearby. Struggling up behind them came old Kirsty (also in her 80s). She always came to the shearing, just to watch.

Fergie had a cardboard box containing some mysterious bottles and three or four old paintbrushes. Paintbrushes? He saw me looking at them.

'Aha. These are for paintin antiseptic on the sheep's skin if the maggots have got to it yet.'

I nodded. The fleeces were thick and any maggots were well hidden. But once the woolly overcoat had been shorn off, they would be visible in the fleece itself, and any damage to the flesh might be in need of treatment. Maggots are pale, disgusting creatures that, if left for any length of time, can burrow into the body of the sheep and virtually eat it alive. It doesn't bear thinking about.

The last to arrive was George – not as fit as the sturdy, hardy crofters who were so used to striding about in the hills. He had in his hand a pair of his own shears, bought for the occasion in the crofters' store in Dalhavaig. He was going to be taught how to use them.

In the 1970s, shearing was still done by hand on most of the more remote islands. They used the large, clumsy-looking, scissor-shaped metal shears that had been around for centuries. Farms in the more affluent south had long been using electric shears, making the job so much quicker and easier. On Papavray, although 'the electric' had come in the 1950s, the supplies were to the villages in the glens, while the fanks, built so long before electricity was thought of, were high in the hills.

More recently, modern amenities have started to become

commonplace. Ugly, galvanised-iron fanks of complicated design are appearing in or near every village, so that 'the electric' is available for the shearing. The old shears are consigned to the back of the byre, and the new automatic implements are used. The collies bring the flock down from the hills to be sheared and then back again.

But today, here on the high hill, there was a flurry of activity, a lot of whistling and soon a group of 20 or so sheep appeared over the brow of another hill. The dogs, who seemed to know by instinct what to do – the crofters giving very few commands – drove the flock into the fank and then lay down at the entrance to discourage attempts at escape. Several men grabbed a sheep each, hauled her into an uncomfortable-looking 'sitting' position, and set to work.

'Right then, George! Tis time you had your first lesson. Y'see, you get hold of her like this . . .' Archie demonstrated as he spoke.

George made a futile grab at a docile-looking beast, lost his footing, and the ewe pranced away. I'm sure she was grinning! After several more attempts, George was ready and Archie handed him the shears. He began . . .

Thirty minutes later, he straightened up, red in the face, covered in sweat and breathing heavily. Then he realised that everyone had been watching him. He glanced down at his poor, patient old ewe. In some places the skin was pink and rather sore, in others tufts of wool stood out like lavatory brushes. A loud, raucous cheer broke out.

'Don't give up the day job, George!' Archie laughed heartily.

George came over to where I was rolling the grubby, oily fleeces.

'Phew! It looks so easy when these guys do it. Five minutes per sheep! My poor beast will probably be psychologically damaged for life.'

'Well, at least you had a go. I wouldn't even get one into position, I'm sure. I'm safer just rolling fleeces.'

Just then, a shout went up. It was time for tea. There was a break before the next batch was brought down from the high hill, so we sat in a circle on the grass or perched on the old walls of the fank and drank thirstily in the warm, bright sunlight.

'Have ye no heard the latest?' Archie was mumbling through a mouthful of dumpling.

'Heard what?' George had recovered his breath.

'About the airyport. Tis to be opened next week, I'm hearin. Some grand body is comin to cut a bit o' ribbon and then the first plane will come in and land.'

'How exciting!' At last, I thought.

'Then it will go off again, takin yon body with it. What's the point o' that, I'm wonderin?'

'It's for explicity,' said Mary knowledgably.

'What?'

'What?'

There was a puzzled pause, then Archie sighed. 'Ach, the woman! I think she means "publicity".'

'Aye,' said Mary, unperturbed as usual.

Archie had been thinking. 'Twill cost a mint, I'm thinkin. The fare, I mean.'

'No,' said Mary. 'I'm hearin that the Island Development Committee is goin to subscribe it.'

Archie nearly screamed. 'Subsidise it, Mary! Subsidise it!' he roared. 'Ach, the woman will be the death o' me, she will.'

'Well, somebody, somewhere is goin to pay something so

that the fares are no too high.' For the first time ever, Mary seemed huffy. Archie looked a bit shamefaced. He had shouted very loudly, and the sound of his voice was still rumbling round the hills.

'Ach, I'd no be so sure,' said Old Roderick. 'I had a letter from the post office last night. It's goin to be about 50 pounds return to Glasgow, they reckon.'

There was a horrified gasp, then Fergie muttered, 'I'm thinkin no one will use it, then.'

'Oh, yes,' piped Mary. 'My sister from Oxford says she will come on the airyplane.'

Fergie sighed. 'Mary, she'd have to get to Heathrow by train or coach, then from Heathrow to Glasgow on the shuttle and then on this plane that's goin to cost a fortune. Very expensive.' He shook his head. 'Better come to Inverness by train and we pick her up from there and bring her by steamer and ferry. Twill be a quarter the price.'

'When is the big opening ceremony to be?' I asked.

'Next Thursday – midday. I hope the weather holds.' Old Roderick sounded doubtful.

Everyone cast worried glances at today's serene sky.

'Hmm,' said Fergie. 'It's been fine for too long. Tis not natural.'

We were getting quite good at reading the weather now, so we squinted with the rest towards the mountains on the other islands, out to sea and finally up towards Ben Criel. Pointing to the herring-bone clouds, Fergie prophesied rain for Thursday. Old Roderick claimed that, as Ben Criel was clear, it might be fine for the great day.

The argument seemed set to continue when Archie interrupted. 'The wireless will tell us.'

Shearing in the sunshine

'Ach! What does the wireless know about Papavray? The steamer canna sail sometimes even though the wireless has said "no gales". What hope has a wee plane? Twill be off more than tis on, I wouldn't wonder.' Old Roderick was lost in thought for a moment, then he said, 'D'ye mind a few years back, ma niece from Canada – her visit? We took her to the mainland for the train to Glasgow for her flight home. Well, we couldna get back to Papavray for the storms. The steamer was off, the ferry had been beached by the high tide, and we had to wait two days. Ma niece, she rang the post office here to say she was home afore we got back. Canada, mind! Thousands o' miles and us just 20 mile away, waitin on the storm. Ach! Twill not do.'

'Well, I'm no goin in one of them wee things. No as big as Archie's boat, foreby. And only six seats!' Kirsty was adamant. 'The only time I'm goin up there is when I die.' She thought about this for a moment and then added, 'If I'm spared, that is.'

I was at a loss to follow this logic, but everyone else seemed to understand.

With that, we went back to our sandwiches and thermoses of tea, happily picking bits of wool off our teeth and lips while the oiliness of the fleeces that I was rolling was likening my hands to something resembling the inside of a car engine. There would have to be a lot of energetic scrubbing before I tended my first patient tomorrow.

'Right! Off we go!' The call to arms went up. It had been decided that the rather protracted tea break should end and the work began again. Another batch of sheep was approaching the pen, so the clipping and shouting and the inspection of the ewes' fleeces and skin continued.

We worked on, glad of the breeze that kept the midges away. George did not repeat his efforts with the shears but helped to bring the sheep down from the high hills. Gradually, the thin, naked-looking sheep began to outnumber the woolly ones. After another three hours or so, the crofters reckoned that they had sheared some three hundred and twenty sheep at least.

'Bound to be a few in the hills that we havena found. Come autumn, they'll be down looking for better grass on the crofts and we'll get them then, but they'll probably have rubbed a lot off and what's left won't be much good. Happens every year.'

Archie was tired, as were all the rest, and they still had to go home to milk cows, feed livestock and shut chickens up for the night. And even continue the hay-making in some cases.

Quieter now from exhaustion, everyone started down the hill, each carrying as many fleeces as possible, tied together in bundles. Just as I had been the first person on the hill, so I contrived to remain behind the once-vociferous crowd as they wearily descended, the tired collies plodding beside them. The uncomprehending ewes, in their white underwear, watched them go and then returned to the important business of grazing.

I sat on the wall and looked out over the green saucer of land that was the village and its crofts. People the size of ants were already fetching in cows for milking and feeding chickens. Gradually, as the peace of the evening settled over the glen, I began to see little plumes of blue smoke rise from the chimneys as folk lit their fires. I listened – even distant voices had stilled, the hill was quiet once more, and I was left in the silent clamour of remembered noise. As the last birds flew off to roost, I picked up my bundle of fleeces and plodded slowly homeward.

Shearing in the sunshine

Home! Our cosy, sturdy, gale-defying home among the tussocky grass, where we could watch the mountains changing colour and shape as clouds, mist, sunlight or even lightning raced between the jagged peaks. Where we had a view of the ever-changing sea: sometimes black and menacing, sometimes silver in owl-haunted moonlight or ice-blue winter sunshine, or, as today, sparkling under the clear summer sky. Whatever the weather or the season, this was a wonderful place to live.

TWENTY-SEVEN

Rowing boats and rucksacks

I gradually came to know the new people who had rented Tin Cottage in Struakin and found Robbie, Sarah and little Fiona to be an unusual and fascinating family. Sarah and I soon found that we had many interests in common.

She and Robbie had left the rush and noise of London, just as we had, but whereas we had to make a living, they had come into a great deal of money, leaving them the freedom to move to wherever took their fancy in order to pursue their hobbies. Robbie was an enthusiastic amateur naturalist, and Sarah was writing and painting and appeared to be very talented.

She and Robbie had been married within a month of meeting. The following year, Sarah had given birth to premature twins. Sadly, the little boy had died and Fiona, the other twin, was brain damaged. While still in London, they had sent her to a special-needs school, but by the time they relocated to Papavray she was able to attend the local school three days a week for mainstream education and was taught at home for the remaining time.

One beautiful day when I was off duty, I drove to the end of the 'road' and set out to walk the two miles of rocky path to the tiny hamlet by the sea. I was hoping to hear that little Fiona had made friends with the Johansson girls. The long school holidays would be very lonely otherwise.

The Johanssons were strange, reclusive people, dour to the point of rudeness. No one knew how they made a living, but Mr Johansson went away for long periods, and it was presumed that these trips were to do with his work. The crofters were curious: he was variously a spy, a scientist, a writer and so on.

Sarah had asked me to tea on this lovely summer day, and we sat in front of the house, gazing at the sea while Fiona played with seashells nearby. The house next door seemed to be closed up although it was unusually warm.

'He's away again,' said Sarah. 'But she is there.'

'What on earth does she do?' I asked. 'Why would she shut herself inside on a beautiful day like this?'

'I sometimes hear a typewriter clacking away but not often. It's the girls that I worry about. In term time, they have other company, but in the holidays they are often inside, not even allowed to play with Fiona some of the time.' Sarah sounded concerned.

'What about friends or relatives? Does anyone ever come to stay?'

Sarah shook her head.

'None of this is a natural life for children, is it?' I said.

'And there is something else,' Sarah said, then paused. 'The other evening at about 11.30 – it wasn't quite dark – Rob was on the cliff with his binoculars. He was watching for a mouse or a mole or something in the bushes beside the shore when he became aware of a movement on the rocks just around the headland. After a while, he saw Mr Johansson leave his house and make his way round the headland. He was going in the direction of the movement that Rob had seen.' She paused to pour more tea.

'This is intriguing – like a thriller,' I said with a smile.

'It gets better. Rob gave up the mousehunt and concentrated on the drama, but once Mr Johansson was round the corner of the rocks he couldn't see him any more. A little later, back came Mr Johansson with a rucksack on his back and went off home. After a bit longer, Rob could hear a very slight noise from the direction of the sea and a small rowing boat appeared, sliding through the water, making almost no sound. He watched, and when it was well out to sea he heard them start an outboard engine and they disappeared into the darkness.'

She looked at me. 'What do you make of that?'

'The most obvious thing would be smuggling,' I said.

We puzzled over this clandestine meeting in silence for a while.

'When did they come to live here?' I asked. 'They were already here when we came.'

'I don't believe they have been here for more than about four years.'

'They have always been a mystery. The crofters would love to know how they support themselves.'

Sarah laughed. 'They must say the same about us, but we are only here temporarily.'

We changed the subject and talked of generalities for a while, but as I started my long walk back to the car I puzzled over the vexed question of the Johanssons. I was concerned for the girls: surely this secretive lifestyle could not be good for them? I determined to speak to Dr Mac. His long experience of people and of island culture made him a wise counsellor who often had a completely different way of looking at things.

In the meantime I enjoyed walking in the sunshine of this perfect day, and I dawdled a little to watch the seals romping in the gentle waves. I listened as I walked and could hear only my own footfall and the song of the birds. No blaring radios, no roar of traffic or honking of horns. No brick walls, high-rise flats or multi-storey car parks. We had left all that behind and this peace was ours!

*

On Dr Mac's suggestion, I began to think up reasons to attend the school more often in order to assess the Johansson girls, but before any progress could be made things were taken out of our hands entirely. And in a most dramatic fashion.

It began with the unusual sight of two high-powered police cars leaving the steamer from the mainland, while John, our own policeman, waited for them on the quay at Dalhavaig in his own modest Ford. The cars were first off the boat and stopped beside John. There was some consultation and then two policemen stationed themselves at the entrance to the quay while John jumped into one of the big cars, which set off at an alarming rate. They roared through Dalhavaig, scattering people and dogs, screamed along the narrow coast road, terrifying sheep and cattle, and leaving goggle eyes and open mouths as they tore off towards Struakin. It must have been a great shock to these enthusiastic young men to discover that they had to leave their powerful vehicles and walk the last two miles to the hamlet.

This was the most exciting thing to have happened on Papavray since the plane crash, but in fact for a quiet, peaceful backwater on the very edge of the British Isles we seemed to have more than our fair share of drama.

Rowing boats and rucksacks

In Struakin, Mr Johansson was arrested and taken away, and, in spite of searching questions, John would tell us nothing. But eventually, of course, we heard the whole saga.

The Johannsons had come to remote Papavray to hide their identity and activities: this was a mistake in itself, as a big city such as Birmingham or Glasgow would have been better. People take less notice of each other in such places than on an island where folk take a consuming interest in their neighbours and newcomers are the subjects of intense scrutiny.

The crime itself was very serious. In spite of all the conjecture about Diarmuid Johansson, no one appeared to have guessed the obvious. This was the early '70s but, although many had decided that he must be a criminal of some sort, no one had connected Mr Johansson with the IRA. Spy, scientist, writer? All these things had been discussed endlessly, and yet the truth should have stared us in the face. Perhaps it was the Swedish name? Or were we just being ostriches about the 'Troubles' because we were so far away from it all?

I heard the story from a shocked Sarah.

Apparently Mr Johansson was heavily involved in raising funds for the IRA. He had organised a system and a route by which money (actual cash) came into the island (the boat that Rob had seen?). He would pass it on when he was on those so-called business trips.

'What about his wife? Was she involved?' I asked.

'I don't think so, but she must have had some idea that something odd was going on. She is the really Swedish one, so she had no loyalty to either side. He is Irish through and through.'

'But his accent?' I asked with amazement.

'All an act, I suppose. Being married to her and having lived in Stockholm for many years, it would probably have been easy.'

'And the girls? Did they know anything?'

'No. They had been told that all the secrecy was to do with "Daddy's work". I have been thinking about her, and I imagine she just wanted to keep the family together. He was devoted to the girls. Can you imagine how a father could help the IRA to blow up families with children just like his own?'

I shook my head. 'It's unbelievable. But what will happen to Mrs Johansson and the children?'

'They are going back to her family in Sweden, I'm told. The house has been searched and emptied, but I don't know any more than that. The police have asked us all sorts of questions, but, apart from Rob's experience that night, we couldn't tell them anything.'

We looked at the view for a while in silence, then she said, 'Rob doesn't want to stay here, and I'm not sure that it is the best thing for Fiona, especially as the girls have gone. So we too will be leaving Struakin.'

So suddenly Struakin would be empty of people and the little hamlet left to the sea and the birds. I hoped that someone would come to live there. A deserted village is a sad sight, and we had too many of them on Papavray.

TWENTY-EIGHT

Peat, trees and trouble

The weather this year had been erratic and the seasons mixed up. On 2 February, George and I had walked to a little coral beach near Coiravaig. We wore thick pullovers and took a picnic, for it was one of those days sent straight from heaven – clear blue sky and silvery winter sunshine. We settled ourselves on the dry white sand and leaned our backs against the rocks, facing the sun and the sea. In no time at all, George was asleep. Oystercatchers romped past, skimming the sea, their red-beaked, black-and-white bodies glinting in the sunlight and their trilling, haunting cry carrying across the water.

June the second saw a snowstorm! The white mantle clothed the far summits for a day or two until a vicious storm and gale-force winds washed it away and we returned to an uneasy spring.

Spring meant skylarks. They were so high up in the dome of the sky that they were scarcely visible and as numerous as 'currants in a dumpling', to quote Murdo, a seven-year-old friend of Andy's.

In April, we watched the skeins of geese flying north to spend their summer in Iceland or Scandinavia, and we listened to the honking and swishing of wings as they constantly changed the leader in their V-shaped formation. In autumn, back they came to share our moors and lochs with the few native geese that stayed all the year.

Another noisy springtime arrival was the cuckoo. No Hebridean cuckoos are ever immortalised in *The Times* by over-eager listeners claiming to be the first to hear that distinctive call. Our cuckoos did not arrive until May, and then Dhubaig alone was alive with at least six mating pairs!

The grass remained stubbornly dormant until about May, when the lengthening days and warmer temperatures stirred it into sudden, burgeoning life. Sheep were let out onto the hillsides, lambs appeared, and people began to look thinner as they shed a layer or two of winter clothing.

As the days lengthened and hopefully the weather warmed, the B&Bs and hotels began to prepare for their brief summer season. The opportunity to make a little money was short lived as our summers lasted for only three months, so the tourists had to be 'caught'. The hotels advertised in magazines in the south – today, they have websites – and put up newly painted signs, while the B&Bs often had ingenious ways of attracting the unwary visitor.

Old Kathy, who lived by the pier, took advantage of this position to stand on the quayside when the steamer was due and approach the disembarking passengers with exaggerated claims about the position and facilities of her small croft house. Sometimes she succeeded in actually escorting them to her rather dingy abode and the more polite among them agreed to stay. But I have not heard of anyone spending more than one night there: they usually found an excuse to move on.

Other potential landladies positioned themselves at the end

of their track where it met the road and waved and smiled until someone stopped. Even if the tourists had only been about to ask directions, they often found themselves politely invited to have a 'wee cup of tea' and then they would quite possibly stay for several days. The average crofters were innately hospitable; they enjoyed the company and hearing about the big wide world, and were only too happy to regale the southerners with tales, often true, sometimes not, of local lore. Many folk thus caught in the crofters' trap would be so comfortable that they might return year after year.

Some visitors, however, found it impossible to understand some aspects of local customs.

By June of each year, great mounds of dried peat appeared beside the road on the high, boggy plateau in the centre of the island where the peat hags are located. The cutting takes place in May, weather permitting, when the crofter wields the peat iron – a specially shaped spade – and cuts the neat shapes, while his wife, or other helper, throws the brown rectangles onto the dry grass, where they look like tidy rows of chocolate brownies. There they stay for weeks, or even months, depending on the rainfall, and when dry are gathered into heaps near the road or track to await collection.

Strangely, many visitors appeared to think that the stacks of dried peat beside the roads got there by magic, and that trees somehow managed to cut themselves into logs, ready for collection. None of these discoveries was deemed to belong to anyone and so were there for the taking. As the district nurse and therefore in uniform, I was in a slightly protected position and was able to right a few of these wrongs. I have to confess that I took a fiendish delight in doing so!

On one occasion, while returning from duty, I saw a smart

new car draw up beside a peat stack. Few island people own new cars, so I knew before I drew near that this car would belong to a visitor. Two occupants alighted and examined the peats. So far, so good – they were interested in something new to them. But then they picked up two peats each, found a plastic bag and, wrapping up their ill-gotten gains, popped them into the boot. I pulled up in front of the car, got out and wished them good afternoon.

I said, 'Forgive me, but have you had the owner's permission to take some of his peats?'

They could not have looked more surprised had I asked if they had the Queen's permission to wear the crown jewels!

After a moment the woman said, 'Owner? Is there one? They were just lying here.'

I explained that they were most certainly not 'just lying here' but were the result of a great deal of hard work and were destined to keep a family warm in the coming winter. Blank faces gradually gave way to a certain sheepishness, but even after my little homily they were not entirely repentant.

'Oh, but we only had a few. That won't make much difference.'

'And when the next car takes three or four and the next and the next?' In spite of its bad roads and its distance from the mainland, Papavray attracted several hundred visitors every summer. Peat stacks would soon be decimated if every passerby took a few peats and this could cause real hardship for some families during the winter. Finally, my victims for the afternoon took the peats from their car and returned them to the stack, but with a very poor grace. I'm sure they thought I was fussing over nothing.

On another occasion, I was driving through our only wood

when I saw another smart little car with the boot open and a middle-aged lady leaning over a wall to receive, from someone on the pebbles below, a huge round log. She staggered to the car and dumped it in the boot then returned, in answer to a shout, as another log was pushed onto the wall by the hidden accomplice. I drew up just as she picked it up. She hesitated as I got out, again in uniform. As with the peat-stealers, I asked if they had obtained the owner's permission to take the logs.

She stood clasping the log, stuttering, 'Why no. I didn't know there was one.'

I peered over the wall. There on the pebbles were several neat towers of cut circular logs looking, with their green lichen, like sliced cucumbers standing vertically on the kitchen table of some precise cook. The crofters often buy a felled or fallen tree, or part of a tree, from the estate, cut it up when they can find the time, or borrow a chainsaw, and gradually take the logs home. This can take months.

In a serious tone, I asked, 'Ah. So the tree felled itself and then cut itself into handy-sized logs just the right size for you to get into the boot of your car?'

Husband had poked his head over the wall by then. 'Oh. I didn't think. They were just lying there.'

Once more, I explained the hard work involved and the system of buying the tree. They were amazed that people could leave logs for months, sometimes years, to await collection.

Then, before he thought, he said, 'But aren't they afraid that they will be stolen?'

I stared at his discomfited face and then at the boot of the car. 'You mean by people like yourselves? But I'm sure these particular thieves are going to put them back.'

They didn't reply. Too shocked at being called 'thieves', perhaps? But they began the laborious task of carrying the logs back over the wall and stacking them with the rest. I didn't entirely trust these two to return all of them, so I unashamedly sat in my car and watched before continuing my rounds.

Are people really so stupid? Probably not. Just entrenched in conditioned thinking: so totally unused to the honesty of island culture that they assume no one would dare to leave anything lying about and that such objects are bound to have been abandoned and so are there for the taking.

I am not pretending that there is no crime among the indigenous population. There certainly is! A very young person may take a jug of milk from a doorstep. There are fights among crofters as a result of too much drink, and we had a persistent arsonist for about two years.

There is also poaching, of course. This is almost a game. Rather like Cornwall's historic attitude towards smuggling, the Hebrides has trouble viewing poaching as a crime. I don't think there was a soul on Papavray who did not have a feast of venison at some time. Even the laird, whose deer they were, knew exactly what was going on within the crofting population. He had a fair idea of which crofters indulged in their 'hobby' but also knew that only a handful of deer would be taken in a year. However, if it seemed that an outside gang of poachers was operating on his land, he would be angry, inform the police and do his best to have the poachers caught and punished. He was not often successful, as it was all too easy to land in the bays, plunder the hillsides and be off under cover of darkness before anyone was aware of the presence of poachers at all.

Peat, trees and trouble

We were too small an island to have gamekeepers as such. The factor and the estate farm manager were as vigilant as possible but the coastline and terrain were rugged and hiding places abundant: even the wind tended to muffle the sound of a rifle shot. Our own island poachers were also vigilant and raised the alarm on at least one occasion. They would not tangle with poaching gangs, however: these people were known to be dangerous and were obviously in possession of guns. But our 'bad boys' did not want 'their' deer taken by outsiders.

I think Duncan was very shrewd. So long as he turned the blind eye, he was in a good position to ask for crofters' help with repairing a boat, catching a horse, doing odd jobs around the castle, dragging a piece of farming equipment out of a burn and so on. It seemed to be an unspoken gentleman's agreement.

So we island dwellers were no saints. But somehow the assumption on the part of some tourists that they can help themselves to whatever takes their eye implies an arrogance that is harder to bear than the 'in-house' peccadilloes.

However, the tourists brought with them a breath of the outside world: new fashions (we only had catalogues), current affairs gossip and much-needed cash. Many were charming and complimentary, and we tried to make them welcome.

TWENTY-NINE

Just another day

One blustery Friday, the two dogs were outside as usual when I heard a frightening amount of barking and snarling, interspersed with yelps of pain. Rushing out of the door, I almost fell over Squeak, who was rushing in with his tail between his legs, while old Bob, Roddy's dog, stood nearby with blood-shot eyes and teeth bared. There was blood dripping from his mouth.

Back inside, it became obvious that this blood belonged to Squeak. He was lying on the kitchen floor with blood pouring from an L-shaped gash on his shoulder. He also had cuts about his face and neck. I was just trying to staunch the flow with a towel when Dr Mac popped his head round the door.

'We were coming to see you. I heard the noise. What have we here?'

He stood looking down at the pathetic dog. There was a sturdy young man by the door whom I knew to be the new locum. Dr Mac was going on one of his rare holidays.

He introduced him as 'Dr Spencer'.

'How do you do's were exchanged, and the young man said, 'Call me "Chas".'

There was no time for pleasantries, however. Squeak

needed attention. Both doctors took a look at the gash in his shoulder and decided that it needed stitching immediately.

'Vet won't be here until midnight at least,' prophesied Dr Mac. 'He's working on the mainland.'

A look passed between them, and Chas went back to the car and reappeared with a bag.

Dr Mac administered a local anaesthetic, and I sat on the floor holding Squeak very tightly to prevent escape, while Chas did some neat sewing. Dr Mac sat nearby and watched.

'Well,' said Chas, as he finished, 'I knew that it would be very different from my Birmingham job, but I didn't realise that the first of my duties would be stitching a dog!'

Squeak healed very quickly and within a month there was no sign of the day's drama, but he gave Bob a very wide berth from then on.

I made the two doctors some tea, cleaned up the kitchen floor and prepared to talk about the patients and their needs. Chas seemed to be more interested in the climbing opportunities than in healing the sick; I think he wanted to climb a hill or two before dark. But he later proved to be most efficient in spite of his easy-going manner.

After they left, I took a cup of tea into the little porch at the front of the house. We had added this when the house was renovated, to take advantage of the view of the mountains. There was only room for two small armchairs, and I sat in one of these sipping my tea and watching the glow of the sinking sun on the craggy rocks, while the restless waves in the bay tossed the borrowed light back to the sky. Gradually, the colours changed as the sun dipped into the sea, leaving a halo of orange clouds and turquoise sky. The hard-edged shadows softened as the twilight – the long twilight of the north –

settled on the glen and the darkened mountains composed themselves for sleep. All was still and peaceful.

But not for long! As I rose to start preparing a meal for my returning and doubtless hungry fisher boys and tired husband, a knock came on the back door.

A neighbour, Ally Beag, stood there, looking uncomfortable. He was not a man that I knew very well, so I was surprised to see him on my doorstep. I asked him in, and he perched on the edge of a kitchen chair. There was a pause, and I sensed that he had something of importance to say, but, of course, we had to go through the usual discussion about the weather, the price of sheep at the last sale and the fishing before he would broach the reason for his visit. Eventually, he offhandedly brought 'Donny the Hill' into the conversation. Donny was an old retired seaman who lived just outside Dhubaig, not far from our home.

'Yon mannie is gettin gie weird, do you not think, Nurse?'

I knew that Donny was becoming senile and had developed an uncertain temper.

'He's no in his right mind, y'know, Nurse. He was on his chimney with the heather in the dark by himself last week, I'm hearin.'

'On the chimney with the heather' meant that he was sweeping his chimney. Usually, with an accomplice below at the hearth, a crofter would ascend the roof, clutching a bundle of heather tied into the middle of a 30-foot length of rope. Holding one end, he would throw the other down the chimney to the person below, who would tug at it, while the crofter on the roof eased the bundle of heather into the flue. Successive energetic tugs would bring the bundle down to the hearth together with vast quantities of brown, sticky soot that would cover the unfortunate helper and everything nearby in a choking cloud of evil-smelling dust. The process of pulling the heather up and tugging it down again would be repeated until one or other was satisfied that the chimney was clean or announced that they would 'surely die of the soot' if they did not stop. The result would be a very clean chimney and two excessively dirty people.

As I listened to Ally Beag, I realised that old Donny was a danger to himself, as this was hardly a job for an arthritic old man at any time of the day, and certainly not alone and in the darkness.

Reading my thoughts, Ally Beag said, 'He ran up and down yon ladder, pullin up and down by himself. He must be 80 if he's a day.' There was a worried frown on his face, and I was beginning to think that the old man might be hurt. I asked Ally.

'Ach. No yet he isna! But that's not all. His dog's no there the now. Nor his cow. I'm thinkin he's made away with them. And . . . ay . . . um . . .'

'Yes?'

'Well, Nurse, it's like this. He's been followin Ida Mackay.'

Ida was a nervous little woman, recently widowed, living in Coiravaig. If Donny were to make a nuisance of himself, she would be terrified. But there was worse to come.

'He has a gun, y'know.'

So here it was, at last! The reason for the visit.

'Aye, well. I must be on ma way.'

And having finally delivered his message, he was off! Half an hour of chit-chat and the real reason left until a second before departing.

I rang John, but I did not want to discuss this on the phone, as the island telephone exchange was a great clearing house for all manner of gossip and this was a decidedly delicate matter.

'I have a little information that I think you should hear,' said I, feeling like a character from a James Bond film. 'It could be urgent. Can you pop over?'

John arrived as soon as the local version of 'popping over' could be accomplished in the deepening darkness, and I repeated Ally's surprising revelation.

'I think I can deal with this fairly easily,' John said, after some thought. 'I doubt if he has a licence for the gun, so I could insist on removing it. If he has a licence, it will be on record, and I'll claim that all guns are being collected for inspection. And then perhaps I can . . . ahh . . . um . . . lose it. If you follow.'

I nodded. 'He is clearly unfit to own a gun. Who knows what he might do with it? That is probably what has happened to the dog and the cow. Obviously, Ally Beag must think so.'

'I'm on my way now, Nurse. Wish me luck!'

And off he went. I did not envy him, but I was so thankful that we had a resourceful policeman who was not bothered about 'following procedures', which might have involved all manner of forms and permissions and delays. Protection of the public 'Papavray style' suited me.

Months later, I was present when we had to section Donny. As far as I know, that firearm is still in John's gun cupboard.

THIRTY

Silent stones and a sad spirit

All over the Highlands and Western Isles can be seen the remains of abandoned villages with their ruined cottages, roofless byres and broken walls. They stand as a monument to one of the most heartless and short-sighted acts of vandalism the British Isles has ever known.

I had read about the 'Clearances', but now that I lived on one of the islands so badly affected I was hearing by word of mouth the stories passed down the generations and I felt the atavistic resentment that still lies smouldering in the hearts of so many. No longer were the people who were driven from their homes merely figures in the history books; suddenly, they became someone's great-grandfather. Now I was meeting big American Scots who were roaming round Papavray looking for 'the old homestead'.

There were several abandoned and derelict villages within a few miles of Dhubaig and we passed one almost daily, but only in winter, when the heather and bracken die away, could one just make out the shapes of the houses and byres. The touring summer visitors never saw such villages: they were long back to their central heating before these old stones made their yearly appearance.

From time to time, I visited another old village by dinghy. Peace now pervaded the remains of this once-thriving township that nestled in a wide, steep-sided valley, running down to the wild sea between heather-clad hills. It was typically placed on sheltered ground, where people could rear their animals, grow their meagre crops and land their fish on nearby beaches. The sea was their only roadway – no tracks ever linked these remote communities. This is Kilcraigie.

One glorious summer day, I pulled my dinghy up the beach and secured it against the rising tide. I tramped over the pebbles and climbed up beside the waterfall. It was a soft, warm day, and I could hear the skylarks rejoicing overhead as I wandered among the old walls, some scarcely visible. The remains of a perimeter wall enclosed the entire village to keep the animals out in the summer, when there was plenty of grazing on the hills, so that the people could grow their precious crops inside. Much later, each croft was separately fenced, but by that time this village was already dying.

I entered the doorway of one house and stood in the room that was now open to the sky. The fireplace, washed clean by years of rain, stared blindly across the tussocky grass, where children once played on the beaten-earth floor. Outside, the byre stood gaunt and useless. No steamy breath of cattle or munching of hay now disturbed this place. The screech of a startled blackbird broke the silence. He soared into the sky and disappeared among the cotton-wool clouds, and the silence surged softly back.

Once this house rang with the shouts of children and the whirr of the spinning wheel. On such a day as this, the men would have been tending their potatoes or turnips. If the summer had been a dry one, they may have been gathering in the hay or the oats. On the beach, all would have been bustle as the one and only fishing boat, manned by the menfolk of several households, came in to land its catch. The burn would have been alive with activity as small children played or paddled, while their mothers washed clothes and blankets, banging the coarse material on the stones and draping them on the bushes to dry. I wonder where they all went? And who among their descendants comes to gaze at the reproachful stones and think of the suffering of those innocent people, on that fateful night, nearly two centuries ago?

*

It was not summer then, with the birdsong and the sun to soften the horror, but a cold, harsh winter's night with snow on the ground and a bitter wind screaming in from the sea, bringing ever more snow. Most of the men were away, as the fishing boat had not made harbour that day; it was sheltering in a cove many miles distant.

Suddenly, the hills were alive with soldiers armed with guns and clubs. They rushed down into the sleeping village, wrenched open doors and hauled the terrified inhabitants out into the snow. Babies were torn from their mother's arms, old women dragged from their beds and dumped outside, while children ran, shrieking into the night. With no hint of mercy, the soldiers threw the meagre possessions outside and set fire to the houses. In spite of the snow, the brittle old thatch soon caught light and within minutes the people were homeless.

The soldiers had long gone when dawn broke and the fishing boat slid into the bay. Huddled on the beach were the fishermen's families, while in the background smoke rose from the blackened ruins of their homes. The men knew why this had happened. They had heard from other boats about townships demolished and families left destitute up and down the coast. They knew that their landlords, Scottish and English alike, had discovered that sheep were more profitable than tenants. With the huge mills of the south demanding more and more wool to feed the hungry looms, and prices rising steadily, the landlords had decided to buy in thousands of sheep. They would roam the hills in the summer, but when winter closed in they would need the shelter of the glens. But the people, paying only a tiny rent, were in the way. So they had to go! Thousands were driven out over the hills or away by sea to who knows where. Some went to the cities, some to far countries, many dying on the way. No one cared what became of them so long as the millions of sheep had room to grow their valuable wool to line the pockets of the wealthy lairds.

What had they thought as they looked back from that tiny fishing boat on all that remained of their lives? I know that life was hard, often lived at subsistence level, but they had a spirit, a determination that took no account of the bare feet and the ragged clothes.

In this denuded glen, there is nothing but silence now, as the sheep, too, have gone.

*

I was brought back from these sad thoughts by a sudden bite on my face. The wind had dropped, so I knew that the ravenous hordes of midges would shortly descend on me in the still air. The midges are the only things about the Hebrides that I detested and resented. We were stoic in rain, resigned in gales, excited in snow and ecstatic in sunshine. But midges . . .

After rising from my seat on the ruined croft wall, I took

one last look around, and while glancing towards the tiny graveyard I was amazed to see that I was not alone! A man in a fawn raincoat was standing beside one of the graves. I started to walk towards him to speak, and, in my hurry, stumbled and fell on the uneven ground. I scrambled up, smiling in embarrassment, as I looked once more towards the man.

There was no one there! The graveyard, the village, the entire glen was empty! With shaking knees, I sat down again. Had he been a figment of my imagination? Or a trick of the light? Or . . .? He had been wearing modern clothes (albeit a mackintosh on a hot day). I could describe his dark hair, his moustache, his down-at-heel appearance and sloping shoulders. I even knew that, in the manner of many raincoats, a fold of material hid the buttons.

After a while, I walked over to the grave at which he had been standing. I looked at the faded and lichened inscription on the rough-hewn granite stone. The sentiment was in Gaelic, which meant nothing to me, but the name gave me quite a jolt.

'Mary Flora Cameron.1804–1840.'

George's mother's family name! I found it all very strange, worrying – frightening even. Was he a lost soul, caught between heaven and earth?

I was suddenly very anxious to leave! My little craft seemed inviting, wholesome, and I chugged gratefully across the sea loch to tie up at Alistair's jetty.

'And where have you been?' The voice was followed by a grubby-looking Alistair, who emerged from a small stone shed.

'Are you all right?' he asked through clenched teeth that were clamped around his ever-present unlit pipe full of dead matches. He peered into my face. He was not a particularly sympathetic person, but now he looked concerned.

'You look as if you have seen a ghost!' he said, with unintentional but staggering accuracy.

At last, I managed to speak. 'Yes, I think you may be right.'

He looked at me with penetrating intensity for a moment and then gazed out to sea.

Finally, he said, 'You have been to Kilcraigie, I gather.'

I stared at him.

'Come on up and have some tea. Alice is in the garden.'

'Yes. Thank you. But how . . . ? Who was . . . ?'

'Not now. Tea first.'

Taking a firm hold on my arm, he propelled me up the 30-odd steps to where Alice was sitting in the garden, wearing her old straw hat and some bright gardening gloves.

'Hello, Mary-J. My word! You look a bit white.' She patted the seat beside her.

Alistair went into the house to make some tea, and I tentatively began to tell Alice about 'the man in the mac', as I thought of him. Sitting in this cheerful, sunny garden beside a friend, I found myself wondering if it all sounded ridiculous. But Alice did not seem surprised or sceptical and nodded sympathetically.

'We have heard about this man before, Mary-J, and many people believe that they know who he is – or was.'

I looked at them. These were two sophisticated, educated people – not some elderly crofters, already steeped in folklore and tales of the supernatural. But they were accepting as fact the appearance of . . . what? A ghost, I suppose.

Alistair was speaking. 'About ten or fifteen years ago, a Frank Cameron came to the island from Glasgow, looking for evidence that his forebears originated on Papavray. I met him once or twice. Scruffy-looking fellow. Stooping. Some sort of university professor. He often stayed at the Ardmartin Hotel, and this particular day he tramped over here to borrow old Ben's boat to go to Kilcraigie. He had some maps and had done some research that suggested that his people might have come from there. The weather was appalling, and Ben was not inclined to let him have the boat. But this Frank Cameron fellow was determined. Said he had to get back the next day to give a lecture and this was the only opportunity he would have. So, much against his better judgement, Ben let him have his boat. Good strong boat. Nothing wrong with the boat.'

Alistair was very fond of the old sea dog who helped him so much with the cruiser. He continued, 'Well, no sooner had this Frank fellow gone than the most atrocious storm broke. The visibility was so bad that we couldn't see whether he reached the other side or not. Ben and I watched for a while, but then we called the coastguard. They couldn't find him. It was three days later that bits of the boat started to come ashore and then they found him washed up on Gull Rock. He was very dead! Poor chap! Only 50!'

'What a dreadful tale,' I said. 'Do you know if Mary Flora was his ancestor? He was standing by her grave when I saw him.' I realised that I was speaking of him as though he were just another person, not an . . . an . . . apparition or whatever. And, indeed, my impression of him had been so vivid, even to those buttons and his tatty old city shoes. Why, I even knew that he had his hands in his pockets! He had been so real.

'You are sure of all this? You're not kidding?' I was suddenly suspicious.

'No, my dear. We can't explain it any more than you can,

but quite a few people have seen him standing in Kilcraigie graveyard. The description is always the same, and that is how he looked when he left here that day.'

Later, when I left for home, I felt depressed and sad, but my sensible side told me that the manifestation was just not possible. But it had happened, and my spiritual convictions were rocking. What could I think? Accept it, maybe, as one of many things that are unexplainable, and say, like Shakespeare's Hamlet, 'There are more things in Heaven and earth, Horatio, than are dreamt of in our philosophy'? Perhaps our philosophy is too narrow. Maybe we will understand one day . . .

George was away, so several days went by before I could tell him about this strange experience. At first, he was inclined to scoff. 'You have been with these crofters too long,' he said. But gradually he began to pay more attention to crofters' tales of weird happenings in general and decided that there 'might be something in this Frank Cameron' after all.

Many, many years later, when I mentioned the 'man in the mac' to him, he was convinced that he had actually seen him for himself. I am still not sure if he was teasing.

Of course, the boys were all too happy to believe me and begged to be taken to Kilcraigie in the hope of seeing 'the man'. I did take them there on several occasions, but Frank Cameron never appeared. I wondered if the boys, for all their bravado, might have been a little relieved.

THIRTY-ONE

Helping hands

One day at the beginning of September, I decided to get the car ready for the winter. This involved packing a spade, a shovel, some sacks, an old piece of carpet and a can of petrol into the boot, while two or three blankets were popped onto the back seat.

September was the month when we began to say goodbye to the glowing green of the bright grass of summer, the joyful birdsong and the long hours of daylight, and anticipate the gale-swept hills and snowy peaks of winter, the big fires and the darker days.

September held the glow of the purple heather clothing the hills and moors: the final swansong before animals and plants closed down for the long dark winter. But some winter days could be beautiful, with glittering silvery sunlight picking out every corrie in the mountains, every white-water stream, and inviting the weary humans to lift their faces to the blessed warmth. Then there was the snow that transformed the winter-weary scene to a fairyland of sparkling majesty in sunshine or moonlight, and young folk screamed with delight as sledges slid and snowballs soared.

Of course we grumbled in the winter (it was too dark and

wet) and in the spring (it came too late and was too cold) and in the summer (when there were too many midges) and then again in the autumn (when the gales began once more). But grumbling is a national pastime, and behind this pretended disaffection with our lot was a deep abiding love for the island, its life, its people and the all-embracing sea.

But we prepared well for the winter. The last of the peats were brought down from the hills and coal was hoarded, as the notoriously unreliable old coal boat began to wallow alarmingly in the heavier seas of autumn. Byre roofs were inspected and made safe, wind-loosened door hinges were strengthened; ditches were dug deeper to take the run-off from the winter rains and chimney cowls were mended or renewed. Without these cowls the down draughts in the beleaguered chimneys would send the thick peat smoke into the room below to kipper the fire-hugging family.

One Sunday morning, I was once again the only car on the road to 'the other side', in this case Cill Donnan. I had the usual daily insulin injection to give to old Christina, who was too arthritic to do it herself. I was sorry for her, but she was an unlikeable lady, being sharp-tongued and derisory, so she was avoided by most of the locals, who termed her 'yon Christina woman'. A ferocious Amazon of a daughter called once weekly to 'do for her', as she put it.

So every morning I chugged up and over Loch Annan to Cill Donnan; I usually had plenty more visits to make but on Sundays she was often the only patient. A round trip of about eighteen miles for one two-minute injection! Not very cost effective, but this sort of thing was repeated all over the Highlands and Islands because our districts were geographically so large.

Helping hands

Suddenly, on a very steep, narrow section of the hill with a drop of many feet to the rocky stream at the side, there was a bang and the little car slewed about, heading for the burn far below. Wrenching the steering wheel over with all my strength, I managed to make her turn within inches of the edge, and she juddered to a halt, broadside in the lane. I sank back in my seat with relief. And then jerked forward again. The steering wheel and the entire steering column had come off in my hands! I sat there for a moment with all this equipment on my lap, utterly astounded.

It was fairly obvious that I had suffered a burst tyre, and I could only suppose that the strain I had imposed on the steering had broken something in the column. So I had a burst tyre and no steering.

Time was passing and I had been late already so the injection was now urgent. This was Sunday, the day when everyone seemed to stay late in bed, so I could not expect help. I decided to leave the car and walk the remaining three or four miles, attend my patient and then look around for some assistance. Leaving a car with a burst tyre and no steering broadside-on in a narrow, steep lane might seem an odd thing to do, but I knew that someone would be along later and would change the tyre and perhaps do something about the steering (I didn't know what was possible), and somehow move it to the side. Such was my faith in the crofters by then!

When I emerged from Christina's dark and depressing croft house in Cill Donnan, there was a dilapidated old car waiting at the gate. A red face beneath the inevitable flat cap grinned at me from the driver's window.

'My, my. You'll be needin a lift then, Nurse.'

'Yes, thank you. You see, I had to leave my car . . .'

'Aye, I know. I saw Dougall, who'd been talkin with Donald, and he'd seen Fergie sortin it. So I came to see were you finished with yon Christina woman and were you wantin a ride.'

'Why, Murdoch! Do you mean that you've come especially?'

'Ach. Tis nothin! No, no, not at all.'

'And you say Fergie has fixed the car?'

'I'm no knowin if it's all right, but we'll see.'

I climbed in and we rattled off in a puff of black smoke.

Murdoch's old car groaned and panted up the steep side of Ben Criel, and there was my little vehicle. The tyre had been changed and the car parked neatly in a passing place.

On inspection, we discovered that Fergie had 'sorted' the steering column back into its housing, found a roll of my sticking plaster and secured it. He had also found a piece of paper and a pen and left a note stuck onto the dashboard with more sticking plaster to say that it should hold to get me home if I was careful.

Murdoch was laughing at the sticking plaster.

'My word! Isn't he clever, just?' After a moment, he added, 'Will I follow you home just in case then, Nurse?'

'Well . . .' The sticking plaster did not inspire confidence, so I was glad of Murdoch's offer. But Fergie was right. It did get me home, and Murdoch came in for a dram, as did Fergie later, and another adventure was over thanks to helpful people.

The more usual companion on my travels on Papavray, however, was Big Craig, Dhubaig's roadman. We were lucky indeed to have such a caring, conscientious man to keep our steep, narrow roads open and the ditches clear. Everyone had reason to be glad of his help at some time. Perhaps none so much as the district nurse.

Helping hands

'Gie me a wee knock if the snow's down,' he'd say. Or if there was a chance of a night call, 'If yon road's bad, gie me a wee knock, or if tis in the night, Nurse.'

Whenever I was called out at night, Big Craig appeared as if by magic. The phone would ring, I would dress hurriedly and, depending on the nature of the call, perhaps ring Dr Mac. Big Craig's croft was near ours, and I didn't even get as far as the 'wee knock'. He would be standing by my car by the time I emerged.

'I saw the lights, Nurse, and I guessed twould be . . .' (Annie/Johnny/Donald/Moira – whoever was expected to die or give birth.)

He'd squeeze his great bulk into the passenger seat, with his shovel and spade between his knees, and off we'd go. Often in snow or ice his weight alone would be enough to enable the car to adhere to the slippery surface and the shovel and spade were not needed.

But it was not only in my capacity as district nurse that I relied on Big Craig. On Monday mornings in the winter, when I had to take the scholars to the steamer for the journey to school, he would be waiting beside the road where it left the village and, with three teenagers in the back, with their week's luggage and books, we would somehow get Big Craig into the front and grind our way up and over the top. He loved these mornings, as he would chat with the boys and tell them about his early life. In company with many of the older islanders, he was intensely interested in the boys' education and plans for the future. Scotland has always worshipped at the altar of education, and the rather exalted title of 'scholar' seemed to me to epitomise this reverence.

Sometimes, it was strangers who helped.

One day, with ice on the road, I turned into a passing place to allow a lorry coming towards me to pass by. I hit a slippery patch and slid gently forwards, straight into a ditch! The lorry stopped and four large workmen, over from the mainland to resurface some roads, came towards me.

Grinning in at the window, the 'gaffer' was laughing. 'Taking a short cut, are you then, Nurse?'

Chuckling heartily, the men placed themselves one at each corner of the Mini and, without waiting for me to get out, lifted the car, with a very startled nurse inside, out of the ditch and onto the road. I thanked them and continued my rounds, feeling as though I had entered some cartoon world.

How lucky we were to be surrounded by so many helpful people!

THIRTY-TWO

The signpost

'Tis gone!' Archie was indignant.

'What's gone?' queried Morag.

'The signpost. I'm no surprised there were nae many visitors at the laird's ceilidh last night. They couldna find their way in the dark because some daftie has made off wi' the sign to the castle.'

There were only two signposts on the island; this one was on the road from our little harbour town of Dalhavaig, where most of the tourists stayed. People for the ceilidh would come from there and would look for the sign, which pointed to the castle in one direction and to our village of Dhubaig in the other.

'No wonder I heard so many cars go by last night,' I said.

'Aye, some folk must have taken the turn for Dhubaig by mistake. They would have a bad shock, foreby, when they found themselves drivin over the Ben in the dark with no ceilidh at the end of it.'

Archie was not speaking of the spontaneous getting together of the villagers for fun and entertainment in the dark winter evenings but of the big organised ceilidhs put on at the laird's castle for the benefit of the tourists, raising much-needed money for the uncertain economy of our small island.

The evenings were drawing in. We were used to driving on our narrow, uneven roads high on the mighty Ben Criel, or between small lochans with the brown peaty water winking at us in the failing light, or peering down to Loch Annan where it brooded far below as we engaged first gear to descend the tortuous track that clung uncertainly to the rocky hillside. But to a tourist, used to double-width roads, white lines, decent tarmac surfaces and street lights for much of their way, the prospect of such a journey must have been daunting in the extreme. And entirely unnecessary, as the castle was in a different direction altogether!

'There's another the night. The last one afore the winter. We've looked all over for that sign and there's no sign of it.' Archie guffawed loudly at his own joke. 'What will we do?'

Mary had been thinking. 'We'll have to destruct one,' she asserted.

We all stared at her. After a moment, Archie gave a long-suffering sigh. 'The woman means construct one.' He turned to his wife, 'Why do you no just say "make" one?'

'Aye,' murmured an unrepentant Mary.

'She's right, though,' said Morag. 'My Angus will make the arms for it. He's good with the wood.'

Old Janet piped up, 'Nay, ma Douggy is better with the wood than your Angus.'

Morag was affronted. 'And what about the letterin? My Angus is better at the letterin than your Douggy. And he can spell "castle".'

Janet bridled. 'So can ma Douggy . . .'

Archie waded in. 'Och! Haud your wheesht, you! Tis only two pieces o' wood: one pointin to the castle and one to

The signpost

Dhubaig. The post is still there, so they can just be nailed to it. It's no difficult.'

Janet and Morag glowered at each other, but I had to leave at that point in the discussion and I just assumed that the matter would be dealt with in the usual way of the Gaels: with heated disagreement but laughing compromise in the end.

Once again, I heard quite a few cars pass that night instead of the usual one or two. Did they not get the sign up after all, so the tourists were still confused, I wondered?

Next morning, as I rattled towards the junction, I could see in the distance two sturdy pieces of wood in place at the top of the post. They were shaped and pointing, one towards the castle and one towards our village.

Archie was standing in the road beside his tractor, looking at the signs. He was shaking his head.

'Can you believe it, Nurse? Those two silly, stubborn old bodachs! They *both* just *had* to prove that they could spell "castle". Just look!'

I looked. The arm pointing to the left read 'To The Castle' and the arm pointing to the right read . . . 'To The Castle'. No wonder the tourists were confused!

THIRTY-THREE

A bonny baby and
some cheery children

On the whole, my work consisted of tending the elderly and chronically sick, administering daily injections to long-term patients such as diabetics, treating others with antibiotics and anti-inflammatory drugs, giving routine immunisations to babies and school-age children, together with dressings of injuries, ulcers, burns and other superficial problems. There were also the advisory visits to mothers of under-fives (no baby clinics here – it was easier for the nurse to visit the home) and frequent attendances at the primary school. Amidst all this work there were the occasions when last offices had to be performed for some departed person or, at the happier end of life, there was the birth of a baby. If these wee souls arrived when expected and not before, they were born in a hospital either on the mainland, if it was deemed to be a necessary precaution, or in the island hospital if we had no reason to expect any complications. Sometimes the 'best-laid plans' went very much awry, as unborn babies do not know the rules.

One October night, the worst autumn storm for many years was raging when suddenly all the lights went out. Such electricity failures were commonplace in winter, but with an open fire, night storage heaters and a Rayburn, we could keep warm and we could cook our food. The freezer was our greatest worry, but like most households we retained all our old blankets with which to wrap the appliance to keep it cool. Just as I had dealt with this, the phone rang.

'Nurse.' It was Dr Mac, and I could tell from his tone that this was no social call. 'Sheena's mother in Coiravaig rang, and it sounds to me as if Sheena is going into premature labour. She's about 33 weeks, I believe?'

'Yes, she is.' I paused. 'We have no electricity here, you know.'

'Neither have we, and it is a rather blustery night. I shall set off now but you should be able to get there much faster, so I'll see you at Sheena's home.'

Rather blustery night! The wind was howling and rain mingled with hailstones like golf balls was lashing down, the sea was a roaring cauldron and Dr Mac called it a 'rather blustery night'.

Gathering my trusty bag, I set off. The little car was buffeted from one side of the narrow road to the other, and where that road perched daringly above the sea cliffs it was not a comfortable feeling. Drawing up to the croft house, which was all in darkness, I spied Sheena's mother, Dolly, waiting in the doorway with a torch.

'She's upstairs, Nurse.'

It was cold upstairs, as, without the electric fire, there was no way of heating the room. But Sheena looked anything but cold. Her face was flushed, and she was frightened and uncomfortable. Her husband, Walter, had planned to be home for the birth but was still at sea, somewhere off the coast of Africa.

'What's happening, Nurse? Am I going to lose the baby?' She began to cry.

'No, no! But it may be thinking of being born a little early. I'm just going to have a look at you.' I was able to examine her by the light of my torch. I patted her hand.

'I think you should just lie quietly for now. Dr Mac will be here in a minute and then we'll decide what is to be done with you.' It was obvious that the baby would be born very soon, and the domestic conditions combined with the power failure were anything but ideal.

As the storm raged on, Dolly dabbed Sheena's forehead with a cool flannel until we saw the flash of the doctor's car headlights.

After a fairly brief examination, he decided that we could not risk having to deliver her in that cold, dark bedroom. Thunder and lightning had been gradually coming nearer. The island hospital was our only option, as it would be madness to get the steamer crew out and toss the poor girl around on a small ship, attempting to get to the mainland. The captain would probably refuse to put to sea anyway in weather like this.

Dr Mac had a large estate car, so we gathered eiderdowns and blankets and made a passable bed for Sheena in the back of the car. Very carefully, she came down the steep, narrow stairs, and it needed the strength of all three of us to stop the fierce gusts of wind from knocking her off her feet. At last, we installed her in the car. I climbed into the back with her and Dolly sat beside the doctor. Sheena was amazingly brave, but it soon became plain that this little baby was going to be born quite soon as she began to moan and the pains started to come more frequently, but it was impossible to time them for the bumping and swaying of the car.

We entered the village of Rachadal, which was all in darkness. The whole island was probably affected, but we knew that the hospital would have emergency lighting. We also knew that it had no incubators. This was a big worry as, at seven or eight weeks premature, the baby would probably be very tiny and ideally would have been better in the well-equipped mainland hospital.

We pulled up outside, several staff came out with a stretcher and we entered the haven of subdued lighting. Sheena was whisked off to the delivery room, where a hospital midwife was ready, so I was free to sit consoling Dolly. Dr Mac reappeared in theatre whites and followed the patient into the delivery room. It seemed no time at all until he was before us once more.

'Well, we only just made it, Nurse! Baby is here! A girl! Congratulations, Dolly. You are a grandmother. I'm going to ring Craigmor and the steamer, and see what the position is to move her on. The child is only 4lb.'

The steamer captain was of the opinion that the storm was abating, so he would get the crew mustered. Then the ambulance driver was called to transport Sheena to the harbour, by which time the steamer would be ready. The roll-on-roll-off ferry (the second sea crossing) was alerted and told of the emergency. Another ambulance would meet the ferry when it reached the mainland and Sheena would be transferred once more to complete her journey. All these people cheerfully left their beds to take Sheena and her baby to safety.

Two weeks later, Sheena was home. Baby Dolleena was thriving and had reached 5lb 2oz.

A bonny baby and some cheery children

Most district nurses, whether in remote areas or conurbations, have a few worrying cases on their books: people who are deemed to be 'at risk'. In the case of children, it is sometimes the health of the child that causes concern, sometimes the environment, and all too often abuse or neglect is suspected. In the Hebrides, however, actual abuse and neglect are most uncommon. The homes are often very basic, the childcare a little haphazard, the food stodgy, the income low, but in spite of these factors I never came across a real case of child neglect or abuse on Papavray. The small homes were always warm where there were children, meals were on the table at roughly the right time, and what does it matter to a child if the chairs are old or the dog sleeps on his bed or if the loo is outside the back door? So long as his parents love him and he has friends like himself, he is usually happy and well adjusted.

But life was not always like that, and I had several people with learning difficulties on my 'at risk' register. There was one family that was a nightmare to try to assist: they were so cantankerous that there was little we could do to improve their lifestyle and squalid surroundings. The mother (I never found out what happened to the father) was now getting old and immobile. When young and strong, she had ruled the house with the proverbial rod of iron because her son and daughter were both 'unfortunate' – a euphemistic term used to cover any condition where the mental abilities were in question. The daughter, Mona, in her 30s, had now to tend her mother, and poor Shona often had no meals or had not been washed or helped from her bed because Mona had gone off and forgotten all about her. The son, Donald, at 20 years old was large and aggressive. Shona had managed him well, but Mona left him very much alone and the neighbours were frightened of him. Oddly, however, he seemed to have an immense respect for anyone in uniform. I was always in uniform when visiting, and even the minister's collar seemed to count, but Dr Mac had to keep an old white coat, left over from his hospital days, to put on before approaching the house.

We all knew that Donald should have been committed years before, but Shona flatly refused. Even now that she was rapidly becoming bed ridden, she would not allow us to place her into a home where she could be properly cared for, because she realised that if she agreed, Donald would have to be sectioned and Mona, she said, would be 'off wi' men'. We tried to keep the volatile situation more or less in hand for several years, but when old Shona died we were forced to have Donald sent away.

Mona did, in fact, 'go off wi' men', as her mother had predicted. Eventually, one of the crofters married her, and we could not decide if, being a Christian, he was rescuing her from her sinful ways or was as crazy as she was. He was very strict with her, to the point of harshness, and we had to keep a very close eye on that situation too.

One of the most enjoyable of my duties was the regular visits to the primary school. The children were a continuous source of interest and amusement. There were about fourteen or fifteen pupils and only one teacher. Mrs Campbell was very popular with her charges and had turned out many a grammar-school entrant, and all this in one room, dealing simultaneously with all ages from five to twelve.

The classroom was cavernous, its proportions causing an echoing resonance. It was heated by a smoky stove and one rather elderly night store heater. For all this, it managed to be a cheerful and welcoming room. The wooden floor was cheered by some bright rugs – the result of craft lessons – while colourful childish paintings adorned the peeling walls.

One lunchtime, I drew up outside the playground and sat for a moment watching the children rushing about. Mrs Campbell, Elizabeth, spied me and came across.

'Ah, Nurse MacLeod! I'm glad of this moment to speak to you. I wanted to tell you, Nurse, that I think Geordie has the measles.'

I was more than willing to accept her diagnosis.

'I'll take him home when I have finished here and have a word with his mother.'

'What is it today?' Elizabeth asked, referring to my visit.

'It's "heads, hands and feet" today,' I said with a smile, thinking of all the none-too-clean little feet, grubby hands and wriggling children. Heads were usually 'clean' – that is, free of 'livestock' – but they had to be checked about once a term.

We had a jolly afternoon with the usual crop of dirty fingernails, whose owners were dispatched to the cloakroom with hot water, soap and nail scrubbers. Feet were often rather smelly through no real fault of the child or their mother but because wellington boots were worn nearly all the time due to the weather conditions. Feet were never cramped or misshapen, as wellies mould to the foot, but as rubber does not allow the skin to 'breathe', athlete's foot was not uncommon.

The children loved to watch each other's hair being inspected, and there was not the slightest embarrassment if I found some 'wee craturs'. Even the child concerned would laugh heartily and depart with me to the washbasins to have their hair treated. They always found fun in the inspection.

'Ach, Nurse, wee Henry's got big fat nits.'

'No, I havenae – they are skinny wee things wi' brown boots.' Laughter at this.

'Ally has mice in his hair instead – there's that much of it, Nurse. Tis a haystack, indeed.'

A good-natured scuffle would ensue. Then, when we got to the feet, there would be more joking.

'Phew! I canna breathe for Archie's feets.'

'Look! There's better tatties than on our croft 'tween Murdo's toes.' And so it went on.

Most of the children were from the same kind of background, their fathers being sailors, fishermen, crofters or working at the pier or the harbour. Their empirical knowledge of the island was most important.

Where was the best place to fish? Where could you see eagles soaring? Who made the best dumpling and was therefore worth a visit? Where was it safe to swim? Roddy had bought a new boat and he might give us a ride to Rhuna. There was a dead seal on the beach that would be worth a look. And so on. Things that mattered in their young lives!

I finished the afternoon's work with a certain amount of regret and gathered up the protesting Geordie to take him home. Even if he stayed away from school now, the damage was probably already done and we might well be in for an epidemic.

THIRTY-FOUR

DIY island style

Living on a remote island meant that many things normally accomplished by professionals or skilled specialists had to be done by ourselves. Painting and decorating, small carpentry jobs, hair cutting, bookkeeping, some house repairs and maintenance were but a few of our DIY 'skills'. But added to these, in my case, were all manner of extras that would not have appeared in any nurse's job description, had there been such a thing!

I had been in twice-daily attendance on a young girl who had suffered from multiple sclerosis for much of her 22 years. It was only due to the devotion of her mother that she was still able to take part in everyday family life, albeit from her bed. Trisha was a pretty girl but due to being so inactive – in fact, virtually static – she had become very heavy. Until recently, her sister had been on hand to help Maggie with the lifting, bathing and bed changing, but she had married and moved away, so Maggie had to call on district nursing care: myself and my relief nurse.

Maggie ran the post office near the pier in Dalhavaig. Her husband, Trisha's father, was away at sea for much of the time, and so the whole burden of the business – customers, mail, pensions, suppliers and so on – fell on Maggie, together with the care of Trisha. She had become exhausted, and Dr Mac had arranged a bed in the local hospital for Trisha so that her mother could have a much-needed holiday. This was the big day.

I was at the post office getting Trisha bathed and ready for the short journey to the hospital – only a couple of miles distant – while Maggie attended to customers.

The steamer was at the quay and would depart in about an hour, and tourists were buying and posting cards before leaving, so that the 'Papavray' postmark would appear on their mail. Maggie also sold little trinkets and 'touristy' things to supplement the rather meagre income from the post office.

At last, Trisha was ready in a warm, red-wool jacket worn over her nightclothes, tucked in a red tartan rug and looking forward to the short ride to the hospital. Ramsey arrived with his ambulance and came trundling up the steep path with the stretcher. Although the house was roughly divided into post office and living accommodation, there was just one path to the only door, so he had to find his way through the preoccupied tourists. After calling a greeting to Maggie, he started towards the downstairs room where Trisha had her bed.

In the doorway, he stopped. I looked at him, wondering what could be wrong: we had done all this several times before for various reasons.

'Hah,' he said. 'Things have changed here since last time.' He looked around the tiny hallway.

I suddenly realised what he meant. Since the last time that we had stretchered Trisha out, some alterations had been made. In order to allow a little more privacy for the family, an inner wall had been built, dividing the already tiny hallway into two parts. One side was the entrance to the post office, which had once been the sitting room of the house, and the other led to the room where we now stood, pondering the situation.

'We'll no get ye round here, Trisha ma girl,' announced Ramsey.

Trisha laughed. 'We didn't think of that, did we?'

Ramsey upended the stretcher and stood it against the wall while he perched on the end of the bed and rubbed his chin. He was concocting a plan. His gaze was on the window: an unusually big one for a croft house. It had been enlarged so that Trisha could see the sea and the garden and even the path to the post office from her bed. She could wave to people she knew, and many local folk dropped in to see her. Pension day was always very busy, and then Trisha had a constant stream of neighbours in to say hello.

I began to study the window myself. 'Is it a possibility, do you think, Ramsey?'

'Aye, it'll have tae be. I'll be seein Maggie for some tools.' And off he went.

I wondered how Maggie would take the news that the whole window would have to be removed. It had a sturdy wooden frame that was cemented into the two-foot-thick cottage wall. There were two opening windows, one at each side, but both quite small, and one large but fixed pane. The whole thing would have to come out. And Ramsey obviously intended to do it himself.

At that moment, Ramsey returned with a worried-looking Maggie. 'Ach. We were stupid, indeed,' she said, and turning to Ramsey she asked, 'Do you think you can get it out in one piece?'

'Aye. I'm thinkin if Nurse holds the windy while I chip the cement away, we'll manage it. We'll stand it against the outside wall and Donald [his son] will come this evening to fix it back in. Do you have the cement, Maggie?'

Maggie laughed. 'No. I have no call to sell cement in a post office.' I admired her placid acceptance of the situation.

'I'll be gettin some from the crofters' store, then.' He paused, frowning. 'It'll have to be on the way to the hospital; the store will be closed later, foreby.'

So it seemed that the nurse, in full uniform, would help remove a window frame and that a bag of cement would accompany the patient in the ambulance to the hospital before being delivered. Nothing surprised me any more!

We pushed Trisha's bed against the far wall, away from any bits of flying cement, and, without waiting to cover carpet or furniture, Ramsey attacked the window with enthusiasm while I hastily retrieved the curtains that were attached to the frame.

We worked on and gradually the frame loosened.

'Hold on to it, Nurse! Tis comin out!'

'Ramsey! I can't hold the entire weight of this,' I cried in a panic, imagining the mayhem if I dropped it. Glass can be heavy and the wooden frame was decidedly chunky.

Ramsey looked at me. 'We'll try to balance it on the sill wall while I nip round to the outside . . .' And before I could protest, he had 'nipped' outside. By this time, my hands and uniform dress were covered in cement dust and my hair had fallen from its restraining bun. We had attracted quite a crowd of spectators, and I must have looked a sight, but I was really past caring and, anyway, the tourists were enjoying themselves, as they had not bargained for so much entertainment! But one large man in a 'toori-bonnet' laughed loudly and so, inadvertently, attracted Ramsey's attention.

Hailing him, Ramsey ordered, 'Come you here and help me!'

A very startled man stepped into the garden and approached.

'Hold here,' he was ordered, and the end of the window frame was thrust into his hands. He was instructed to take the weight and 'no drop it'. Ramsey then nipped back inside to take the weight from me and we began pushing it towards the man outside. It was now more than halfway out, so Ramsey nipped outside again to join the man, who, beginning to enjoy his adventure, called to his family to take a photograph 'fert chaps in't factory at 'ome'.

Between them, they manoeuvred the window, amazingly intact, onto the ground and propped it up against the wall. I was thanking the weather gods for the balmy, sunny day. I could imagine only too well what the scenario would have been in our usual gales.

I popped upstairs to wash my hands and dust myself down, and when I returned I found Ramsey, still covered in cement dust, placing the stretcher beside Trisha's bed. Maggie briefly left her customers to help us to lift her daughter onto it.

'How are we to get it onto the window sill – if you can call it that?' I wanted to know.

Maggie chipped in, 'I'd like to help but look at yon queue! And the steamer's gettin ready to leave, so they'll all be clamourin to be served.'

'Get you back to them, Maggie,' said Ramsey. 'We'll manage.'

I looked at him with horror. I'm quite a strong person, and obviously well used to lifting patients, but the idea of the two of us trying to lift a sixteen-stone girl onto the window hole, through it and down the path to the ambulance . . . well!

'Nay, dinna worry, Nurse.' Ramsey winked and cocked his head. 'We'll make them work for their entertainment.'

He turned towards the window hole. 'I want three strong men,' he bellowed to the gaping crowd.

There was some shuffling, and then three men detached themselves from the throng and approached, grinning sheepishly. Ramsey marshalled one man to hold one end of the stretcher with him and instructed the other two to hold the other end.

'Now, when I say "lift", you LIFT,' he ordered. 'We'll put her on the wall [the sill] and then gently push her forward about three or four feet. Then we [he indicated the man beside him] will come round and take this end again.' He looked at the men's rather dazed faces. 'Clear?'

They nodded wordlessly.

Under Ramsey's barked orders, the rather involved process was completed and all four men eventually stood outside, one at each 'corner' of the stretcher. Trisha was enjoying every minute! Taking full advantage of the press-ganged help, Ramsey marched them all down the path and into the waiting ambulance, carrying the stretcher. I followed with Trisha's possessions and made her comfortable.

We thanked the helpers, who trotted off to the waiting steamer. It transpired that Maggie had rung Rhuari and asked him to delay its departure, and everyone had been happy to oblige. What a tale the tourists would have to tell when they arrived home!

Maggie came out to say goodbye to Trisha. She'd go to see her in the hospital before leaving tomorrow.

'Donald will be here after work to put the windy back.' Ramsey looked around. 'We made a wee mess, didn't we?' he remarked.

Maggie sighed. 'What's worrying me is how are we to get her back in again if Donald puts the window back?'

Ramsey slapped his head. 'I'd no thought o' that! But, indeed, we canna leave it all open.' He pondered. 'Oh well, we'll just have to do the same thing all over again.'

And with that, he climbed into his ambulance, we all waved to Trisha, and off they went to the hospital. But presumably to the crofters' store first for the cement!

THIRTY-FIVE

Echo House

So another season was coming to a close as we left September behind. Not for us the sudden mass exodus from hotels and B&Bs the weekend before the schools started their autumn term. Our tourism was not primarily based on families with school-aged children. Many of our visitors were retired or early retired folk, who toured from hotel to hotel throughout the Highlands and Islands in the comfort of a well-sprung car. When they got to Papavray and her neighbouring islands, they certainly needed the springs! Because many folk were unused to passing places, there were many dented bumpers and some serious crashes, but Archie earned a lot of pocket money pulling cars out of ditches with his tractor.

Other big groups to descend on the island in all but the very worst of the winter weather were the climbers. They were usually students on long vacations from university or beginners being led and taught by large booming professionals in yellow jackets. Our Ben Criel, although steep and tortuous, was only about 2,000 feet and was probably ideal for the beginners.

Even so, accidents happened. Every year, there were at least two tragedies among the various islands that made up the

Western Isles. It was not unusual for gloom to settle on Papavray as yet another enthusiastic young man tumbled to his death on our rocky hills.

Papavray could only accommodate about thirty people comfortably at any one time in the hotels and B&Bs. Some hardy souls pitched tents when and wherever took their fancy, while many stayed with friends or relatives on the island.

There was one building on the island, however, that did not fall into any of the usual categories for holiday accommodation. It rejoiced in the name of 'Echo House'. Not so very many years ago it had been an old bothy with an attached barn, perched in a dip in the hills high on the side of Ben Criel. The brave couple who now lived there were not locals. Brian (Bri to everyone) and Dij (I never found out what her real name was) had been climbing on Papavray one summer some years ago and had been unable to find anywhere to stay. In most mountainous regions, climbers are housed in hostels, but there was nothing of that nature on the island. Brian and Dij realised that they had found a gap in the holiday business and they set about with a will to fill it. They both gave up jobs in the south, and Brian rented the bothy, improving and extending it. Incredibly, they opened for business the very next spring and were immediately inundated with enquiries. The next year, another bit was added, and the same thing seemed to have been going on every year since.

It was not palatial. It did not pretend to be. Brian and Dij knew that climbers needed and expected only the bare essentials: comfortable beds for weary limbs after a long day's climb, masses of good food to fuel the same limbs for the next day and somewhere warm to relax in the evenings and to dry their clothes and boots. The couple also knew that they needed to keep the prices down, as most climbers were young and impecunious. So the bothy's interior walls were still of rough stone, the heating was by huge peat fires, cooking by a second-hand (maybe fourth- or fifth-hand) range, lighting by oil lamps and the toilets were 'out back'. There were two dormitories and one or two double rooms, all with bunk beds. Brian had knocked two of the downstairs rooms together to make a farmhouse-type kitchen, and everyone ate together round a large wooden table. The place was a Mecca for climbers!

There was always a happy if rather frenetic atmosphere in Echo House, and those two people worked harder than anyone I know, but I never heard a complaint from them about the workload nor from their visitors about the primitive conditions: only praise for the friendly welcome and physical comforts.

But here again, the cruel world did not pass them by. I suppose it was inevitable that as most of the island climbers stayed at Echo House this was also whence most of the casualties came. Unsurprisingly, Brian trained and joined the mountain rescue team, and many of the unfortunates were brought back to the hostel. The injuries were often serious, and one year alone there were two deaths from Echo House. A sad end to two young lives.

Echo House? How did it get its name? Exactly as one would imagine. You can stand at the front of the building and shout whatever comes to mind and your voice will return to you from the surrounding hills not once, not twice, but several times until it dies away like the final notes of the 'Last Post'. A truly unearthly experience.

Whilst filling up with petrol at the garage, I bumped into Dij, and as this was a rarity we decided to brave the draughts (and the coffee) of the pier 'café' to have a chat. We chose a table by the window so that we could see the steamer leaving. But this was no ordinary departure.

Dij and I watched with sadness as a group of soberly clad men and women followed a coffin onto the boat, doubtless bound for a resting place many miles away. It was, once again, a young man from Echo House who was now making his last voyage, and Dij had driven his friends here.

Dij was a motherly soul who felt these losses deeply. Some of the youngsters had been coming to Echo House for years, so she knew them well.

'Only 22,' she murmured. 'He had married since the last time he came and his wife – widow – is pregnant.'

We were silent for a while as we watched the ship slip quietly away from the quay and steam off.

Dij sighed. 'I suppose it's not all gloom,' she said. 'We do have fun and romance and terrifically interesting people to stay.'

'Very hard work, though,' I ventured.

'Oh, I don't mind. I wouldn't want it any other way.' She paused. 'Shall I tell you a funny story?'

'Anything to cheer us up would be good,' I suggested.

It seemed that a few weeks ago Dij had been in the kitchen when the knocker (a huge piece of driftwood that Brian had found on the shore) thumped on the door. She happened to be wearing a cooking apron that had been bought for Brian to wear when washing dishes. Brian is about 6 ft 5 in. and 16 stone while Dij is less than 5 ft and rather plump, so as she answered the door she must have looked a bit like an animated tent. She had been taken by surprise: in an isolated spot like Echo House, you do not expect 'droppers in'.

On the step stood the most beautiful girl in the whole world (Dij tended to exaggerate a little). Tall, very slim, blue-eyed with shoulder-length blonde hair, this vision was beautifully made up and exquisitely dressed in a smart black suit and court shoes. This was so unusual that Dij just stared for a moment.

'Hello,' said this apparition in a rather deep, musical voice. 'I am afraid I haven't booked, but do you have a room for a few nights? I have some unexpected time off and I wanted to complete my list, you see.'

Dij was used to these 'lists' for, rather like the Munros, there were a number of mountains on various remote islands that had to be scaled in order to hold one's own in certain climbing circles.

Recovering slightly from shock, Dij noticed all the climbing equipment on the ground beside this smart lady. She explained that they had no rooms available at the moment but she could find a bunk in a dormitory. To her surprise, in view of her guest's sophisticated appearance, this willowy creature seemed quite happy with this arrangement. Feeling shorter and fatter by the moment, Dij led the way up one of the two staircases. She threw open the dormitory door and stood aside.

But instead of entering, this vision of beauty stood looking at the sign on the door, which clearly read 'Women's Dorm'. Dij looked at her enquiringly, thinking that perhaps things were too spartan for such an elegant person.

The rather melodious voice said, 'Ah. I'm sorry. I should have explained. I like to dress like this sometimes, but I really need the men's dormitory!'

Dij's jaw nearly disappeared into the voluminous apron. 'You . . . you mean you're . . .' she stuttered.

'That's right,' came the confident reply. 'I'm a transvestite. Is there a problem?'

'Well . . . um . . .' Dij had not met a transvestite before.

'Oh, I know what you are thinking,' the happy voice continued. 'You think I'm gay and that I shall cause trouble, don't you?'

'Well . . . um . . .' Dij had no idea how to deal with this situation.

'No, no. I'm not gay. These are my wife's clothes. I just like to wear them sometimes. It's a bit of a lark, really. Now, do you think I might have a cup of tea when I have unpacked?'

Dij and I laughed until our sides ached.

'How did it go?' I asked, as I finally dried my eyes.

'He turned out to be the life and soul of the party. He had a lovely baritone voice and we had some great evenings. He was an accomplished climber too.' She paused. 'It takes all sorts, I suppose.'

And with that, we parted.

THIRTY-SIX

To the rescue!

It looked as though winter was starting early. Outside was a veritable winter wonderland. Huge snowflakes were dancing in the light breeze and floating gently to the waiting earth. The hard shapes of the rocky outcrop beside the house were softened to rounded hillocks, while snow crept up the windowpanes from the sill below and the fence posts wore jaunty white hats several inches thick. Our home-made track to the house looked unbelievably smooth: the only time that it looked smooth at all was in the snow!

The real beauty of this virgin scene, however, was beyond the garden. The mountains were starkly and pristinely white, except where the peaks were too sheer for the snow to settle, and granite cliffs rising vertically from the sea looked naked with their steep sides shining wetly in the glaucous light.

The ruin of the old church on the shore resembled something from a fairy tale as its walls were coldly cushioned by the falling flakes, and the few remaining snarling gargoyles began to look ridiculous, rather than frightening, as they acquired snowy wigs. The village was becoming amorphous, as croft boundaries, pathways and gates disappeared. A few cattle stood about, heads low, breath visible in the cold air.

'I think I will go and fetch Sunshine. I won't be able to feed her in the morning if it snows like this all night,' I said to no one in particular. George was watching a programme on the flickering television, and Nick and Andy were hoping that the snow would get deep enough for sledging.

Although the pony's field was less than quarter of a mile distant, the track to it was so steep that it might have been impassable by morning, so it seemed wise to bring her to the tiny paddock by the house while I still could.

I trudged off through the deepening snow, and as I neared Sunshine's field I was surprised to see Iain-Angus, our vet, wandering around the shore in an apparently aimless way. But our vet was never aimless! He was a very hard-working man: up at 6 a.m. and often still tending some sick animal at midnight. In fact, if we needed him for one of our animals, we sometimes had to wait until the early hours, as he served several other islands as well as an area of the mainland.

He saw me and raised his hand in greeting, continuing to walk along the beach. A walk on a beach in a snowstorm was not a normal pursuit, I thought.

'Iain-Angus! What on earth are you doing?'

'I might ask you the same thing,' he said with a grin, glancing at the white heavens.

'That's easy. I'm going to get Sunshine to take her to the house,' I replied. 'But what are you up to?'

'I think I'm wasting my time, Mary-J. I had word that Dhubaig's Commission bull was in trouble somewhere here. I came straight here, but with this snow I canna see well. He's a big fellow, though, foreby.'

'Perhaps he's over by the cliffs?' I offered.

To the rescue!

The vet peered through the curtain of snow. 'Mary-J. Look! Can you see? Is it himself?'

Over on the rocks was a dark shape, only visible because all the rest of the surroundings were white. I glanced at Sunshine. She could wait for a little while, I decided.

'I'll come with you,' I shouted to the retreating figure of the vet as we both started to flounder across the beach. All the while there was a little nagging thought at the back of my mind. This is a bull. He might be injured. He might not be pleased with life.

Iain-Angus read my thoughts. 'I'll see what's wrong first. You stay back a bit.'

The island bulls were free to roam, and with plenty of 'wives' to keep them busy, they were usually very docile. But it wouldn't do to be too complacent.

I could see that he was lying half on his side among a tumble of large rocks, and as the vet approached he raised his head and 'grumbled' in his throat. Iain-Angus bent down beside him, and it was apparent that one leg was caught between two of these big boulders. Going to his head, the vet tried to encourage him to rise in the hope that the movement might be sufficient to release the leg, but the animal seemed unable to respond at all.

'He's well and truly stuck. I don't think there is anything broken, but he's been there some time.' He indicated a pile of dung behind the bull. 'I think he has exhausted himself trying to get out.' He stared out to sea. 'It must have happened since the last high tide, but it will be back again in less than three hours. We will need to get him out very soon.'

He stared at the trapped animal for a moment. 'Right. It will take three or four men to move the rocks, hold the bull and so on. I can't sedate him if he's to help himself to get up, so it might be dangerous. He must weigh a ton or more.' He rumpled his shock of greying hair. He never wore a hat or cap, even in weather like this.

I was thinking quickly. 'Suppose you stay with him and I run Sunshine home and get some of the crofters? Would that help?'

'Aye. Indeed. Archie and his tractor, Fergie, Murdo . . . perhaps Donny. Lots of rope, some crowbars. Yes, yes. And some sort of halter . . .'

'I have that,' I interrupted. Sunshine's halter would be too small, but I knew Iain-Angus would manage somehow.

The vet continued, 'I'll stay and try will I prevent him from struggling any more. Off ye go then, Mary-J! Perhaps George . . . ?'

I left him mulling over the problem. I collected Sunshine and we trotted off side by side – it was too slippery on the hill to ride her.

Once home, I shouted the news to George, and after handing Sunshine over to Nick I rushed off over the croft to find Archie while Andy ran to tell Fergie, thinking that this was even more exciting than sledging! I knew that I did not need to fetch anyone else, as all the activity was bound to be noticed, the reason quickly relayed, and plenty of help would be forthcoming.

Archie was soon coaxing the cold engine of his ancient tractor into smelly, belching life. Fergie appeared with Andy, both carrying sizeable pieces of rope, and down the hill came Murdo and Roddy, complete with two hefty crowbars. Everyone seemed to know by ESP what was needed. Soon, a small army of men were plodding through the snow.

I gathered a few first-aid bits (not for the bull: I felt that we would be lucky to get away with this little endeavour without human injury). Alistair had popped in to say hello, and it was lucky that he was here because he had a vehicle that we all called the 'Thing'. It was a conglomeration of bits from an old tractor, part of a pick-up truck and various other weird cogs and wheels that Alistair had fashioned together to pull his boat up the beach. It was high off the ground and because of the snow he had come visiting on it. He called it 'Hilda'!

When told of the problem, he took his pipe out of his mouth to say, 'Let's go! Hilda will be useful, I'm sure.' And off we went, Andy and I riding on an incredibly uncomfortable 'Hilda'. The snow clouds had gone and a watery sun was trying to warm the shivering shore.

Iain-Angus was still crouching beside the bull, trying to stop the animal from hurting himself further.

'Come here quietly,' he called to the advancing mob. 'He'll get edgy if we all rush at him.' The crowd stopped a few yards away.

'Now,' said Iain-Angus. 'If a couple of strong chaps can gently get the crowbars into the gaps between these rocks . . .' He indicated the gaps in question to Murdo and Roddy, who had gone forward. 'Can we have the two vehicles ready nearby? Tie the ropes to them. We might need them to help heave him up when he is freed.' He looked round, and the precise instructions continued until he was satisfied that everyone understood their position and what they were to do. Nick, Andy and I were told to keep back 'in case'. Alistair was on Hilda, ropes at the ready, with George beside him to assist. Archie was nearby on his gently chugging tractor, while Fergie together with Donny (young, strong and fearless) stood near Iain-Angus.

'Mary-J, you keep an eye on yon box [his veterinary equipment] – I'll maybe need that when we get him out. Now, everyone, if his injuries allow, he will be off the minute he is released. Be ready to get out of his way! If we can catch him, we'll take him to Mary-J's horse shelter for me to look him over.

'Right. I have the halter. Roddy and Murdo – you are ready with the crowbars. Fergie, Donny – you will grab his horns. Try no to move too fast.'

The horns in question were long and sharp, so, although he was big and black, he must have had some 'Highland' in him somewhere.

I suddenly thought. 'Does he have a name? Would he respond to it?'

They all looked at me as though I had grown two heads.

'Well, the cows often know theirs,' I said in self-defence. 'I thought it might help if he did.' They all thought I was mad.

Iain-Angus rescued me. 'He has, as it happens, but I doubt he knows it. Tis "Boris".'

There was silence. A bull that has been given a name like 'Boris' is unlikely to be a quiet, docile creature. We all eyed him with misgiving, and I wished fervently that I had not asked.

'Right, we are all ready. Let's go!'

Everyone leapt into action. Roddy and Murdo edged forward and, with one eye on Boris, inserted the ends of the two crowbars under one of the rocks, while Donny and Fergie gingerly leaned over the vast shape of the animal and grasped his horns. He immediately tried to raise his massive head, but the two men held him firmly and the vet took this opportunity to slip the halter in place. As the first rock eased, Boris attempted to move his trapped leg, but the second rock still held it firmly.

To the rescue!

As the men wedged the crowbars under the second rock, Iain-Angus motioned to everyone to be aware that the animal would be free at any moment. The rock was moved away but, although he struggled, Boris could not rise.

'He's been there so long I'm thinking he's stiff and cold,' said the vet. He motioned for the vehicles to approach slowly. With the rocks now out of the way, Roddy and Murdo threw down the crowbars and joined Fergie and Donny to keep the thrashing bull still while the vet managed to get the ropes round the huge neck.

'Get you behind him and push to get him on his feet when the ropes are taut!' The vet addressed the men holding the bull still. 'When I say, start pulling!' This was to Archie and Alistair on the two vehicles.

After a moment – 'Now!'

The two vehicles started to move away and the ropes tautened.

Another 'Now' from the vet and the four men behind the bull started to heave and push while the ropes pulled steadily. Iain-Angus was pulling at his head and murmuring encouragement. Boris began to scrabble with his legs, trying to raise himself. His own efforts, in addition to the pulling and pushing, gradually began to show results. First the back legs and then the front gradually found purchase on the slippery rocks and he was up.

'Watch you now!' Iain-Angus warned, but Boris was too wobbly and dazed to be any threat to anyone. The vet unhitched one of the ropes from the bull but left the halter and the other rope round his neck and started to walk him away from the rocks onto the snowy sand.

Calling over his shoulder, Iain-Angus said, 'Turn off the

engines and follow me on foot, in case [in case of what, I wondered]. Mary-J, bring the box and someone go ahead to open the gate to Sunshine's field, and I'll need something strong to barricade the entrance to the shelter. [The horse shelter was open, with no door or gate.] I can see a sizeable gash on his leg from the sharp rocks.'

Our little cavalcade set off, and once we were well away Archie took off at some speed on his tractor.

'He'll be fetching a door or something for the shelter,' was Fergie's opinion.

Into the field we went. Boris seemed very quiet and biddable. Now that I could appreciate his full size, I realised how brave these men had been to tackle such a notoriously unpredictable creature as a bull, and a frightened bull in distress at that! Iain-Angus was leading the animal into the shelter, turning him so that he could see the leg more clearly.

'Hold his head.' He handed the halter to Fergie and bent to peer at the leg. As soon as he touched it, Boris threw up his head in protest.

'Hmm. I'll need to give him a local. The box, Mary-J, if you please, and perhaps another two of you to help Fergie and Donny? He will not care for the needle.'

And he didn't! It took the combined strength of all the men to hold him still, but gradually the local anaesthetic took effect and Iain-Angus was able to do a little fancy stitching to a four-inch L-shaped gash. Nick and Andy gave Boris some of Sunshine's hay, and he munched happily during the whole procedure.

'Right,' said the indefatigable vet. 'Now we need something to keep him in here so that he does not rush about and start the bleeding or pull the stitches.'

As though on cue, the unmistakable sound of Archie's old

tractor was heard, and he swung into the field. He had attached his trailer and on it was a large, heavy wooden byre door.

Nick and Andy and the rest of the men helped him to unload it and place it across the opening. Archie had brought wire, hammer, nails and small bits of wood, all of which would now be used to secure the door for the night.

'Just remember to let Iain-Angus out first,' laughed Alistair.

'Where did you find this?' asked Fergie, looking at the door with suspicion.

'Ach, it was just lyin around,' muttered Archie.

'I recognise it. Tis that one Kirsty got from old Dougall the Hill for to mend her byre. I'm surprised she let you have it. She's been waitin on young Barry to fix it.'

'Ah, well . . .' Archie looked a bit sheepish. Fergie stared at him.

'She didn't let you have it, did she? You just took it!'

'Ach. She'll no be out in this weather, foreby, so she'll not be missin it. I'll have it back long before that good-for-nothin nephew of hers gets round to fixin it.'

No one was hurt during the dangerous rescue, and we all trooped home to warm up and dry off. The bull recovered well and in a few days was wandering the hills, doing his 'duty' again.

The snow melted almost as fast as it had fallen, as so often happens in the islands, and Andy and Nick did not get much sledging done. But the excitement of the day made up for that.

THIRTY-SEVEN

'Arry's island

One bright, sunny day, I sat on a low, rocky hill near the castle. The wind was gentle and the sky was a deep blue with odd grey and white clouds shaped like buns and some like saucers. I could see why folk sometimes claimed to have seen a flying saucer. In a poorer light, these clouds scudding by were a remarkable shape and could so easily be mistaken for an alien object. I could not, however, see anything resembling the little green men that seem to figure so highly in fiction. Why 'green', I suddenly wondered?

A small boat was chugging its way towards the shore below my rocky perch. There was the tiniest of harbours tucked between two outcrops of rocks, and in bad weather it must have taken great skill and nerve to negotiate the narrow entrance. But today the little craft glided safely into the sheltered space on clear, calm water. A grey seal circled the boat several times before deciding that it was not likely to yield nourishment; he could not smell fish on board, so he swam away to find lunch elsewhere.

A slight, rugged-looking man landed at the tiny quay. He sprackled up the slope towards me.

"Ow do! It be a grand day,' he called.

'Hello,' I replied, trying not to show my surprise at the accent. It was Cornish! Now here must be an interesting tale. He didn't give the impression of being a tourist, so what was a Cornishman doing in the north of Scotland?

He plonked himself down on the ground beside me. ''Ow be thee, then, maid?' he asked chattily. We exchanged views on the weather, the castle and the state of our little world, but I was consumed with curiosity. It must have shown.

'You'm wondrin what a body like me be doin yer. Well, I'll tell 'ee.'

And he did! He introduced himself as 'Harry' – or 'Arry. He had been a soldier in the Second World War, and his company had been sent to the Faeroe Isles to provide a deterrent to enemy attempts to blow up supply ships taking the northern route and to thwart any attempts to invade Britain from the north.

Harry told me how the men were welcomed into the communities and, like so many of his compatriots, he began to get friendly with the young Faeroese girls. He became interested in one quiet country girl called Olga. The young folk fell in love, and after the war Harry returned to marry her and settle down on the Faeroes. But being unskilled, he found it difficult to get work, try as he might. Harry, a farmer's son, had only ever worked on the farm until war drew him away.

While he was in the Faeroes, his father died and left him the farm in Cornwall. Olga took some persuading to move from the isles of her birth and from which she had, so far, never ventured, but Harry could really do nothing else, so they eventually moved the thousands of miles to the very southern tip of England.

'Ahh, twer the only thing to do. But she weren't 'appy. No.

'Er din't say much, but I knew. Ah, I knew.' Harry shook his head and a sad expression came over not only his face but seemed to spread to his whole body. 'But she put up with it fer some years. She missed 'er family and the long summer days of the North. 'Er couldn't get used to the warmer weather in Cornwall and she missed snow in winter.'

'I would have sent her back for an 'oliday now and again, but I couldn't afford it. The farm 'ad been 'it with foot and mouth, and the cattle 'ad bin slaughtered. The compensation were pifflin and we was strugglin. Olga were pinin fer 'ome and I din't know which way to turn. 'Er were in some state!'

But evidently fate took a hand when a letter arrived from Olga's brother in the Faeroes. He had been working on the oil rigs and had made a great deal of money, so he, Sven, had now fulfilled a long-held dream of leasing the small remote Hebridean island of Ardnacloich.

'I know it,' I said, thinking of Jaynie and Baby Janet. 'It forms part of Duncan's estates.'

'That's right. Clever man was Sven. Knew what 'ee was about all right.'

'Anyow, 'ee wanted me to go and work for 'im on this 'ere island. Twas about three miles long and two wide. No electric, but a wind generator, and no ferries or anythin. Just you and your own boat. Well, Olga were ecstatic. Twas North again, y'see. Not Faeroes, no, but same sort of place and climate. And 'er brother were married to Sonya, 'oo 'ad bin 'er school friend. Ahh! Twere an opportunity at just the right time.'

Harry sold the Cornish farm, and he and Olga set up home on Ardnacloich. It seemed that the venture was a great success. The two couples got on well together and many fulfilling years went by. Although so far north, it was sheltered by the Outer

Hebrides, so they grew just about all their own vegetables and even some fruit. They kept sheep, goats and cows for food and to sell. Buyers had to travel to the island to purchase their chosen animals, Sven and Harry being unwilling to leave their beloved isle.

Harry's enthusiasm faded a little as he said, 'Olga was all right because 'er brother and Sonya were there, but I don't think 'er 'eart were in it as much as the rest of us. 'Er 'ad to work some, but I did as much as I could to save 'er. To make sure 'er were as 'appy as possible . . .'

He sighed. 'I've come to go up to see this 'ere Lordship. 'Ee never comes to the island. Says Sven looks after all the books and such like so well that 'ee's 'appy to leave us be. But now . . .'

He sighed again. 'You see, we'm goin to 'ave to leave Ardnacloich dreckly. Sven and Sonya drowned a few weeks back. Twas a right tragedy, it were!'

I murmured my sympathy. I could see what was coming.

'Olga and me, well us couldn't manage by ourselves. With all the animals and the land. I couldn't expect Olga to do too much, but I 'ad wondered if we coulda got a coupla lads to 'elp but 'er din't want to carry on. Sven 'ad left the lease and the money to 'er so we could've afforded to do that, but no, 'er 'ad 'ad enough and it's 'ers now so . . .' He sighed.

I offered him a lift to the castle, and he clambered in.

'So what are you going to do?' I prompted him.

'Well, us made friends wi' some folk from 'ere, who come to Ardnacloich to buy some goats . . .'

'Goats?' I interrupted.

'Ahh.'

'There is only one croft on Papavray that has goats. So it must have been Fergie.'

296

'Right. And another fellow. Archie were 'is name. Cousin or something.'

'Well! I am surprised. I remember the goats coming, but I didn't know where they came from. They are very handsome animals.'

'Ahh. The best! Us only breeds the best.'

'So, what are you going to do?' I repeated.

'Well, this 'ere Fergie said as 'ow I should come and see 'is Lordship and see if us could get an 'ouse and work 'ere.' He seemed less than enthusiastic.

'Tis more convenient yer. You got some shops and tis better fer getting to the mainland and so on. Olga would like that.'

'Where is Olga just now, by the way?'

'I left 'er in Dalhavaig and come on round meself. 'Er 'ave to see some solicitor 'bout the money Sven left her. Do you know 'im? Angus Mac-something? Is 'ee all right, because I 'opes 'ee's straight with 'er?'

Angus was the only solicitor on Papavray. 'Yes, I know him. He will be straight with her.' What I felt I did not need to say in these circumstances was that if there was ever something very private, local folk went to a solicitor on the mainland. Angus could be talkative.

But I was beginning to see that this likeable little man had spent most of his adult life trying to make sure that Olga was 'all right' and ''appy'. I was also forming a picture in my mind of a small, rather clinging little woman with blonde, Scandinavian-type colouring, who needed a lot of care for some reason. Maybe her health was delicate? She had not wanted to leave the Faeroes with him, had not been ''appy' in Cornwall and now was looking forward to leaving Ardnacloich. I had heard nothing of what Harry wanted. Did they have to give up the lease? Surely they could obtain help, because men were always looking for work and there was precious little around.

We pulled the old-fashioned bell and the big heavy door was soon opened by Chrissie, who now worked for the laird.

'Chrissie! This is Harry, who has come to see Duncan.'

'Hello, Harry. The laird is expecting you.'

Just at that moment, Duncan exploded into the room in his usual boisterous manner.

'How do you do, Harry?'

'Well. Thank'ee, sir.' Harry was ill at ease. Duncan, although friendly, could be a little overpowering.

'Come through, Harry. We'll go into the study. I have a few ideas that might interest you: a possible future for your island.'

'Thank'ee, sir, but tis Olga's island really, because it's her lease now, ain't it?' Harry was hurrying after the laird. But Duncan suddenly stopped and looked round at Harry.

'No, no. The lease was in the name of Sven Polson. Now that he is sadly no longer with us, it reverts to me, to reassign as I see fit, as part of my estates.'

And off he strode, with Harry almost having to run to keep up. I just heard his receding voice saying, 'Well! I weren't aware o' that, sir. I thought . . .' And they were gone.

Chrissie beckoned me, and I followed her into the vast warm kitchen, where a kettle was singing on the Aga.

'Tea?'

'Please, Chrissie. How is young Johnny? And what is happening now?'

Chrissie was busying herself with tea, and dumpling, of course.

'He's gone back to Gran and Gramps, as he calls them, for

now, to finish school. He's very clever and might be a vet one day. He goes to see Biddy, but . . .' Her face clouded. 'It upsets him, but he still goes. Indeed, he's a good boy. When he comes to see her, he stays with us for a whiley, so we are getting to know him.'

She beamed, and we settled down to drink tea and gossip: a very agreeable pastime! I had said that I would drive Harry to Dalhavaig to join Olga.

After a while, an unusually quiet Duncan came looking for me, followed by a very subdued Harry. I didn't understand the changed atmosphere but rose to take Harry on his way.

'Thank'ee again, sir, all the same. Tis good of 'ee and I be sorry 'bout this. I am not ungrateful, sir. No, I ain't.'

'Well, well. Just talk it over with, er, um . . . Olga, and I'll hold everything in case . . . Ah, yes. Yes,' Duncan humphed and his voice trailed off. 'Yes, yes, Harry. Talk to er, um . . . Olga, and come back to see me if you feel that you can go ahead.'

'Thank'ee, sir. I'll do that.'

Farewells were made, and Harry and I departed.

'Well,' he said. 'That there lordship be very kind, very generous, but I don't think Olga'll go fer it. No, 'er 'eart's set on 'ere or more likely the mainland. 'Er's lost interest sin 'er brother died.' He paused for a while, chewing his lip. Then, with a sigh that came from the bottom of his boots, he continued, 'I sometimes wonder if 'er woulda stayed there wi' me at all if it weren't fer 'im.'

I let him ramble on. It seemed that Duncan and the factor had come up with an innovative idea for the future of the island and, with it, a future for Harry and Olga. It could be run, said Duncan, as a sort of 'summer school' or 'outdoor-pursuit centre'. Young people could learn animal husbandry and crop management. Added to this could be facilities for naturalists and even for painting holidays. Harry would teach animal husbandry and would be in overall charge.

In his usual endearing but blundering way, Duncan had forged ahead with these ideas with ever-increasing enthusiasm, and for a while Harry was swept along with growing excitement. This was just what would suit him and a wonderful way to ensure the future of the island that he had come to love so much. But gradually he became quieter. He didn't think Olga would be ''appy' doing this. She was nearly 50 and didn't want to work any more. She had Sven's money and didn't feel she needed to. Again, I wondered if what Harry wanted had entered the equation at all. He, too, was only about 50 and not ready for pipe and slippers.

It was a very dejected Harry whom I drove into Dalhavaig to join Olga. He looked around.

'She'll be at the quay. Ah. There she be, in that there café.'

We pulled up outside the damp and dreary harbour café. Harry waved and out came Olga. At least, I assumed it must be Olga, but where was my mental picture of the delicate little woman with Scandinavian colouring?

Standing there, with arms akimbo, was a tall, hugely overweight, dark-haired virago of a woman, who immediately began to berate Harry in a loud, hectoring voice.

For a moment, I was in shock. So much for preconceived ideas! This was the woman whose happiness had dictated Harry's every move for his entire adult life. He tried to introduce us, but Olga pointedly ignored me.

Diffidently, Harry began to tell Olga about Duncan's idea. As I turned away – obviously she did not want me there – I caught sight of Archie, Mary and Fergie standing nearby, watching the scene. Fergie unobtrusively lifted his arm and beckoned me. What now, I wondered?

'Come you here, Mary-J,' said Archie, and drew me a little way off – out of earshot of Harry's pleading tones and Olga's grating, accusatory voice.

'Yon woman! You know Fergie and I went to their island back last year to get his goats. Well, we both took to Harry – a nice wee mannie – but yon woman was not around, so we didn't see her at all. From the way Harry talked, we thought she would be as nice as he was.' He shook his head. 'Fergie heard that Harry was comin to see the laird about the island now that Sven Polson is dead,' he continued.

Fergie took up the tale. 'We thought we might bump into him, so we were waitin here by the quay for him and we saw him bring her here. He just landed her and went off again, but it was obvious who she was. We couldn't believe it! Great big, bad-tempered-lookin lump of a woman she was.'

'Yes,' I said, wondering where all this was going. 'She had to come to see Angus about the money that Sven has left her.'

'Aye, we know,' said Mary. (Of course they knew!) 'Angus came out after she had gone, and he was mutterin and moppin his head. We all went for a dram, and Angus told us all about it. Angus said that she stamped and swore at him. Aye, she swore at him when he told her that Sven had left the money jointly to Harry and her, not just to her as she had thought. And she had thought she had the lease now. To sell! Stupid woman! Everybody knows that it re . . . rev . . . goes back to the laird.'

Fergie now continued. 'When she finally calmed down, she demanded her half of the money there and then. Thousands!

He rang the bank and off she went, stampin away to get it. We saw her.'

These three had been busy!

'I'm not knowing what Harry is plannin with the laird, but, whatever it is, she'll not be a part of it.'

'What do you mean, Fergie? "She'll not be a part of it"?'

'Y'see, we had a wee bit shoppin to do, so we sort of followed her up the road. Guess where she went!'

'Where?'

'Back here to the Steamship Offices!'

I was stunned. A dreadful suspicion was beginning to form in my mind and in the next breath Fergie confirmed it.

'I followed her in, pretended to be lookin at some brochures. You know what? She booked a one-way ticket, single, to the Faeroes. She's leavin him!'

I looked across at Harry and Olga. They were quieter now. She was standing in a triumphant posture, Harry just standing. Shocked? Distressed? Or . . . what? Unsurprised, perhaps?

As we watched, she strode off towards the hotel without a backward glance. Harry stood looking at his boots for quite some time. I believe I thought that he would watch her go or call out to her, even run after her. He did none of these things, just stood looking at his boots with a deep frown on his face. After quite a few minutes, he raised his head, took a deep breath, braced his shoulders and began to walk towards us. In that moment, he seemed to have grown in stature, determination and confidence.

Nodding to Fergie, Archie and Mary, he addressed me. 'Nurse . . . will you take me back to that there Lordship, please? I b'lieve we can do business after all!'

THIRTY-EIGHT

Old folks' secrets

One December morning, I was telling Mary about our plans for a visit to London as she sat beside me in the car.

'Aye. Twill be good indeed,' she replied. 'And will you be going to all yon big shops, like Harrods and Belfridges?'

'Selfridges? Yes. Harrods? No, too expensive!'

'Aye,' Mary pondered. 'I'm thinkin I'd not like London at all. Too expensive and too many red buses. I've seen them on the television. And they have the Underground too! Why do they need buses and Underground? Can they no make up their mind?'

'There are so many people in London, Mary, that they need both methods of transport to get them all to work and then home again.'

'So why do they no live nearer to their work? I'm not understandin these London people at all.'

'Houses are too dear in London, so most people commute.'

'What is that?'

'They travel in and out of the city.'

'Mmmm.' Mary was obviously not convinced. After a silence of a few minutes, she returned to more familiar topics. Local ones.

'You'll be goin to see old Sara, no doubt?'

'Yes. She is getting so odd and forgetful that I'm afraid we'll have to send her away for her own good eventually, but she has lived in that house all her life, I'm told.'

'Aye, but she's getting that weird. It's the coal now, I'm hearin,' rejoined Mary cryptically.

'The coal?'

'Aye. She's polishin the coal now.'

'Oh my!'

Old Sara, now at 85, was very odd indeed. She had always been inclined towards excessive cleanliness. She used to wash the cows' faces, brush the sheep and attempt to comb the chickens' feathers when she ran her parents' croft. Now we often saw her polishing the windows with furniture polish and sweeping the grass by the door. Inside, everything shone, either with furniture polish or Brasso, and the old-fashioned range was black-leaded daily. Her clothes all had a bleached look from so much washing in harsh soaps and chemicals. More recently, she was becoming a danger to herself. I had found her walking in the snow in bare feet one day because she did not want to get her shoes dirty. On another occasion, I treated some infected scratches that she had sustained from the sharp claws of her bad-tempered old tomcat when she had decided to plunge him into a tin bath full of soapy water. When I remonstrated, she said, 'But he was dirty!' Now, it seemed, she was polishing the coal!

I knocked on Sara's shining door. Receiving no reply, I peeped inside. A waft of furniture polish greeted me.

Sara was crouching before the fire in the old range, piling peat and coal onto some crackling sticks. She glanced up as I approached. 'Ah, Nurse! Tis you. I'm just gettin a good blaze here.'

She was! The well-polished coal, with several lumps of polish still adhering to it, was spluttering and sparking, and, as she claimed, a 'good blaze' was roaring up the chimney.

But Sara was standing too close! The edge of her voluminous skirt suddenly caught light.

She screamed and started to beat at the flames with her bare hands.

'No! No, Sara!' I grabbed a cushion from the couch with one hand and tried to thump the skirt, while trying to rip it off with the other. The cushion (probably well polished) caught light immediately, but the skirt was coming down and off easily, as it was only held up by elastic at the waist.

'Step out of it, Sara. Step out of it!'

But Sara was rigid with her mouth open, still screaming. She was tiny, so I picked her up and pulled her free of the blazing skirt and dumped her unceremoniously on the couch. Still she screamed. But I had to deal with the fire.

There was a bucket of water in the corner. I dowsed the burning skirt, the cushion and the rag rug that had now begun to smoulder. I threw all the black mess outside and turned my attention to Sara, who was still screaming. I talked to her, I touched her, I shook her; the screaming continued unabated. I splashed cold water in her face and eventually and very gradually the screaming stopped, her mouth closed and she relaxed against the back of the couch. At last, I was able to look at her burns. Her hands were tough and work-worn, so there was only slight redness, while her legs had not been affected at all. Perhaps the thick black stockings had protected her. At least they did not appear to have been polished!

'What about ma skirt, Nurse?' She struggled up and was making for the door. 'I have to get ma skirt.'

'It's gone, Sara. Burnt! There is nothing left. Have you another?'

She ambled to the box-bed against the back kitchen wall. Kneeling down, she began to rummage beneath it, pulling out all manner of bits and pieces: trinkets, tools, a bridle and bit, and finally a thick, sack-like garment that she held up in triumph.

'This is ma other skirt,' she said, pulling it on over her petticoat.

It was green with mildew, but Sara did not notice and squeezed herself into it. It was much too tight. She looked most uncomfortable in this child-sized skirt. Child-sized? It couldn't be, could it?

The next minute, Sara confirmed my almost rejected thought, by saying, 'Aye. I wore this when I was a wee girl – for school, y'understand. Tis a good strong skirt!'

'Yes, Sara, it is strong, but it is far too small for you now. Do you have another?'

Sara appeared to think for a moment. 'Aye, I have. But I'd no like to spoil it.' And she wandered over to a big trunk in the corner and began to struggle with the lid. It was obvious that it had remained closed for many years, but between us we eventually prised it open.

I gasped as I peered inside. Sara was pulling out the most gorgeous royal-blue satin dress, much embroidered and bejewelled. I could see more beneath it: shiny silver lace, gold satins, red velvets. So many beautiful fabrics were all carefully folded and stowed in this battered old trunk.

'Y'see why I'd no like to spoil it by wearin it?' Sara held it up with pride. I judged the style to be from about the late 1800s. There were frills and flounces, lace, a tight bodice, a big skirt and a low neckline. It had probably been intended as evening wear for a wealthy and fashionable lady, and I had a little difficulty in imagining Sara wearing this to lock up the chickens for the night or fetch in the coal.

'How did you come by all these lovely things, Sara?'

'Aye. Twas ma mother. She worked for Lady Leticia Briggs – her that married yon laird in the big house on Lewis that's fallen down and I'm not surprised. Lady Leticia gave her all these when she married. Ma mother, that is, when she married my father. She never wore them, and then she left them for me when she passed over. I have to look after them for her, y'see.'

As Sara spoke, she shook the blue dress she was holding and a cloud of dust joined the smoke still lingering in the room. But the dress could not withstand this treatment and began to break up. Bits of lace dropped to the ground, and the sleeves began to come away from the bodice. Sara looked on in horror.

'Look, Nurse! Tis fallin to pieces. Oh, what would ma mother say? Oh dear, dear!'

Huge tears formed in the old eyes and ran down the smoke-grimed cheeks. 'Ach. I'll be puttin it back. Twill do for to dress me when I go to meet ma mother.' She looked at me. 'You'll do that for me, Nurse, won't you?'

I felt a sense of shock. It would be hard to say why, but I think it was to do with her complete and unquestioning belief that she would see her dead mother soon and that I would be here to dress her for that great journey. I assured her that I would do what I could when the time came. What else could I say?

The next minute, Sara had forgotten the dress and all that it meant and was bustling about. 'I'll be cleaning up all this mess and then I'll get ma grate black-leaded.'

I could do no more and left, determined to call tomorrow with a skirt of my own that I had ceased to wear. She was much smaller than I was, but with the addition of some waist elastic it would be fine and it would be a good excuse to see what she was up to the next day. I worried for her safety.

Here we had the usual dilemma of the elderly when they became confused and forgetful. They were usually perfectly happy in the family home, in which they might well have been born. But they were often a danger to themselves with regard to fire, falls, electricity and sudden illness. So, was it better to leave them where they were, happy but in danger, or insist on removing them to some sort of care, where they might be physically safe but quite possibly miserable? The eternal problem.

As I walked along the quay to my car, a voice hailed me.

'Nurse! Tis good that I have caught you,' Behag called from her doorway. 'Tis old Neilly.'

'Sorry?'

'Neilly! He's gone!'

'Ah.'

Behag shuffled her feet a little. 'You'd best see Maggie afore you go to him.'

'Yes. I know about Neilly's circumstances, Behag. Dr Mac and I have tried to get him treatment and care again and again, but he wouldn't have it.'

'Aye. Maggie told me.' She paused. 'You'll be goin there now, Nurse?'

'Yes, I will, and I know only too well what I shall be dealing with there.'

'She'll be waitin there, outside the house. She saw your car at Sara's.'

I drove the short distance to a little copse beside the road. Through the overgrown trees and bushes, a narrow path led to the dilapidated croft house. The thatch was patched with bits of tin, the door propped up with a piece of wood, while thick brambles obscured the walls and windows. The place was a sad sight.

Maggie was standing outside, whispering with two crofters. 'Ah, Nurse. Tis a bad do, this.' She was pale and her face had a wide-open, shocked look.

'Maggie.' I touched her shoulder. 'You found him?'

'Aye, I was making a try would he let me in to give him this.' She indicated a cup of soup that she still held. 'He usually shouts at me to go away. Ach! But today there was no sound, so I peeped round the door. And there he was. I didn't go near, Nurse, but it was obvious that he had gone – a long time before.'

Poor Maggie. She was the only person who had been able to get near the old man for weeks now. Neilly had known for months that he was dying of cancer but stubbornly refused all efforts to hospitalise him or arrange care and medication at home. Dr Mac had tried many, many times to reason with him, but even when he was in excruciating pain he refused drugs and would accept no treatment of any sort.

Even before his illness, he had been a sour, grumpy old man. Even Dr Mac received the sharp edge of his tongue, which was something unknown on the island, as the good doctor was beloved by all. In spite of Neilly's surly ways, everyone had tried to help him in the terrible months leading to his death. If ever a death was a blessed relief, this was the one.

For years he had lived a hermit's life, only emerging to pick up the food and milk that Maggie delivered to his door. The money for these meagre requirements was left in a bucket outside. We were aware that he never washed his clothes or himself, or cleaned his home. He did no repairs of any kind, went nowhere and saw no one, slipping outside only to gather peat from his dwindling peat stack or coal from a huge heap delivered several years earlier. How he spent his time in his dark, malodorous house, we never knew.

For the last four or five days of his life, he had been unable to leave his bed, even to use the stinking bucket in the back porch. (Until then, a nearby crofter had emptied this receptacle weekly into his own cesspit.) Maggie had continued to brave the smell and the tantrums to leave glasses of milk or soup by his bed. So I was all too aware of the state in which I would find the deceased.

'I'll bring you some old rags and towels of mine, Nurse. They can be thrown out afterwards. And I have an urn of hot water ready that we'll bring over. And some soap. I'll bring a sheet too.' Maggie set off.

I pushed open the door. The smell was overpowering and I actually retched. Pulling myself together, I waited for my eyes to adjust to the gloom and then made my way to the window. With much effort, I was able to open it, poke my head outside and take a deep breath. Only then did I look at the bed.

Poor Neilly must have died in torment as well as in filth. His face and his limbs were contorted, his eyes were staring, and one hand clutched the soiled sheet. I was appalled. Why had he refused help, care, ease from pain?

I approached the bed with care. The rotten wooden floor was full of holes, some so big that a whole section had fallen down and now rested on the mud below. The bed was at a crazy angle, and one corner was held up by a concrete block. The room was bitterly cold and damp, having had no fire for many days.

As I was putting my plastic apron and gloves on, there was a tap on the door. Maggie handed me the urn of hot water, the towels, rags and a crisp white sheet. I took these from her and prepared to turn away, but she said quietly, 'Nurse, you have the window open.'

I had forgotten the rule in island culture that while a 'corpus' is present, all doors and windows must be kept securely shut.

'Maggie, I'm sorry, but I can't work in here without some air. You know what the smell is like.'

'I suppose not,' replied Maggie. 'Aye, well.' I realised that I was flouting tradition, a thing I normally tried hard not to do.

'I'm sorry,' I said again. 'I promise to shut everything tightly when I have finished.'

'Right. I'll have some hot water for you to have a good wash in my house, Nurse, when you have finished. And then a nice wee cuppie, perhaps?'

'Thank you, Maggie.' I had obviously been forgiven.

I think there is no need to go into details about the next hour. It will not be difficult for the reader to imagine the state of the patient after four or five days unable to leave his bed and unwilling to allow anyone to wash or help him in any way. Suffice it to say that, with one horrendous exception, it was the worst service that I have ever had to perform for a patient, alive or dead. But finally poor Neilly was cleaner in death than he had been for many a year in life and, wrapped in the crisp white sheet, he finally looked at peace. I paused for a moment when I had finished, to pray that he was now in a better place than this awful hovel.

I shut the window, did what I could to secure the door and

then took the urn back to Maggie. She had the bathroom warm and the water hot, and I gladly washed and scrubbed myself before drinking the much-needed cup of tea.

Maggie said, 'You can ring Roddy [the undertaker] from here.'

'It's all right, Maggie. I'll ring from home.'

Maggie looked at me. 'Nurse, you should ring now so that he can get here before dark.' She glanced at the clock. 'It's near three now.' But I still did not appreciate the urgency.

She continued firmly, 'Roddy must remove him, Nurse, in the next hour at the outside. Because of the rats.'

I went cold. Rats! Of course! Many of those holes in the floor were not from rot but from rats. And you cannot leave a corpse where there are rats. What a dreadful scenario that conjured up.

'Maggie, of course! I still have a lot to learn.' She smiled sadly and handed me the phone.

But the story did not end there. When I went to inform Dr Mac of Neilly's death (of course, he had already heard), he opened a drawer in his vast old-fashioned desk and withdrew two envelopes, one slim and one very bulky.

'The last time I went to see Neilly to try to persuade him to allow us to treat him, he was a little more inclined to welcome me. Well, not exactly "welcome", but he handed these to me. I was to open the fat one and read its contents but not tell anyone about it until his death, when I was to open the other one.'

'What are they?'

'The small one is a kind of will. He leaves everything to Maggie . . .'

'But what on earth did he have that Maggie could possibly want?'

'This,' said the doctor, picking up the larger packet. 'It is Neilly's life story. His spidery writing is not easy to read and his grasp of English grammar is poor, but I'm quite sure that a publisher would be interested if it could be typed out and tidied up.'

Dr Mac settled back in his chair. 'Briefly, he was born on Lewis, the oldest child of a brutal, drunken father and a mother who committed suicide after the birth of her fourth child, who was malformed. Neilly was literally the "whipping boy" of the family. If the father beat him, he left the rest alone for some reason, so Neilly put up with this treatment to protect the other children. His father was in and out of prison, so Neilly, only a boy himself, brought up the three younger ones. They had very little money and none of them seem to have had much schooling, but eventually they grew and left. Neilly joined the army and saw action in several theatres of war, including the Second World War. He was captured, starved and beaten.'

'I saw the scars,' I murmured.

'Aye, and from his father, I wouldn't wonder,' rejoined the doctor, who then continued this harrowing tale. 'After the war, he went to the States, joining the New York Police Department. He married and had a son. His wife and son were both killed in a drive-by shooting. He blamed himself, as he believed it to be a reprisal because he had been the means of bringing some big-time gangster to justice. He came back to Papavray, to his uncle's croft, a bitter man, resolved never to love anyone or trust another soul as long as he lived. His story stops abruptly when he became ill, but it would have been the end anyway, I imagine, knowing the sort of person he had become. His hermit-like lifestyle would not have yielded much of interest for his pen.'

Dr Mac finished speaking. I remained silent for a moment, thinking of this terrible story.

'So this is what he was doing in that dreary hovel. We did him an injustice, didn't we?'

'We couldn't know,' said Dr Mac.

'But I still don't understand why he would not accept any help and drugs when he developed cancer?'

'I wondered about that.' Dr Mac shook his head. 'I think he saw it as justice – a rightful punishment. As I said, he blamed himself for the death of his wife and young son.'

'Poor man! Poor man,' I muttered.

Dr Mac took a deep breath and straightened up as though throwing off the gloom.

'Now this needs typing out.' He looked at me, speculatively.

I left to drive home, thinking about the day. Poor Neilly, with his terrible life and dreadful death, and old Sara slipping into dementia. Apart from the kindness of neighbours, they were both alone and unloved at the end. For all its beauty and gentle way of life, Papavray had its sad side.

THIRTY-NINE

John and Joanna

My eldest son John was unable to spend much time on Papavray because he started working at an early age. Never one to enjoy school, he found college 'boring', he said. He left after only one term and found a job in a huge antique market. He loved the buzz and excitement of London. He shared a flat with some friends and enjoyed the independence and freedom of this pulsating city. Now, many years later, his one desire was to find a home with no buzz, no traffic and no crowds. But he wanted more sunshine than Papavray could offer.

We knew that he had met a girl in London. Her name was Joanna and it seemed no time at all before they moved in together. This was not as common in the '70s as now, but we had to accept the arrangement as John was 19 and Joanna 20.

We had no sooner come to terms with this news than John rang to say that the antique market had closed and they were both out of a job. Optimistic as always, he was not worried as he would soon get something else, he said.

The weeks passed and we heard nothing. He had no telephone and was the world's worst correspondent, so we just waited to hear how they were faring. One evening, the phone rang.

'Mum.'

'Yes. John! Lovely to hear from you!'

'Mum, are you sitting down?'

That question always meant trouble! I sat suddenly on the stairs.

'I am now. What's wrong?'

'Mum, Joanna's pregnant! Can you find me a job and somewhere for us to live on Papavray?'

What a bombshell! I was very glad that I was sitting down. I was lost for words.

'Mum? Are you there?'

'Yes . . . What are you going to do? I mean . . . are you . . . ?'

'We are going to stay together and bring up the baby . . .'

'When is the . . . ?'

'April.' A silence.

'Are you going to get married?'

'Well, perhaps. We hadn't thought about it.'

Another shock! Papavray was old-fashioned – 30 years behind the times. This would not go down well. I turned my attention to his requests.

'I can probably find you a job of some sort, just to start you off here. When you have been here for a while, I expect you will find something else for yourself. Somewhere to live will be more difficult, but I'll try. A caravan is about the only thing I shall be able to find, I think.'

'Please try, Mum. We are a bit desperate as we've no money, or not much. I need a job badly. I'll ring in a couple of days.' A pause. 'Mum?'

'Yes?'

'Thanks.' The pips went, signalling that he'd run out of money, and he was cut off.

For a while, I sat where I was, looking at the phone. John – out of work – no money – a pregnant girlfriend – hadn't thought of marriage – needing a home and a job on Papavray. It was a lot to take in. It was as well that he had told me to sit down!

The first thing was to send him a cheque and then ascertain if there was work and accommodation to be had. And, amazingly, it was easy. Two days later, I had found a residential caravan for rent in Dhubaig. It was a bit basic, but they could take showers at our house and do their laundry in my machine. It so happened that the captain of a lobster fisher was looking for a deckhand and, although John would have to be away for three or four nights a week, the work was available immediately and the wages quite good by Papavray standards.

John rang. 'Great, Mum. Thank you. We'll be there the day after tomorrow. I've bought an old banger from Gerry. You remember Gerry?'

I did – just. But he was part of a different life.

'Will Joanna be happy about the caravan, do you think?'

'It can't be worse than this miserable hole. See you soon.'

Two days later they arrived. A few clothes, some blankets, a number of personal items and quantities of tools and spare parts for the 'banger' were packed into a battered minivan.

Joanna, a pretty girl, was a decided shock to Dhubaig, with her flowing dresses, headband and carpet shoulder bag. She rapidly added an old Afghan coat and some workman's boots to this startling ensemble.

After they had settled into their caravan and eaten an enormous meal with us, John lost no time in going to see the captain of the *Silver Fish* – certainly fishy but far from silver. He was a man of drunken habits and uncertain temper, but

John was 'set on', to start at 4 a.m. the following Monday, the Sabbath being safely over.

I tried to spend some time getting to know Joanna. Although they seemed very happy together and she was coping with her pregnancy well, it became worryingly obvious that she was a city girl at heart, and I wondered how she would deal with the quiet isolation of Papavray. And a more personal worry was whether the notoriously fraught relationship between mother-in-law and daughter-in-law – or as near as – was going to work. We were so different! I thought of myself as a very ordinary wife, mother and district nurse. Joanna was a colourful hippy, or free spirit, with an intolerance of the ordinary and a rejection of all things traditional.

John hated the job and was not sorry when the captain ran amok one night and was arrested. No one knew what was to happen to the boat, so John promptly left to look for other work. He became an estate worker for Duncan's farm manager and was much happier; he was also home every night, so Joanna relaxed and began to enjoy the island. They moved to a bigger caravan in Cill Donnan and started to make friends, so I was cautiously optimistic about their future together on Papavray. After all, we had done much the same thing ourselves: abandoning everything we knew in the south and coming to the island, and we did not regret it for a moment.

FORTY

Days of ice and fog

It was the sixth day of the great freeze! The cold air seemed to ignore the presence of eiderdown and electric blanket, and seeped into the bed so that I was almost glad to leap up and rush below to huddle by the Rayburn. The boys were there before me, as were two dogs and two cats. No one wanted to move from the warmth, but even the Rayburn, that traditional bringer of comfort, was sluggish in the windless, freezing air. There were no teasing gusts in the flue to coax life into the reluctant coals this morning. The night storage heaters had been set to 'high' for days, but the cold was so intense that they only warmed a few feet of space around them.

Wet and windy we could manage; this intense, all-pervading iciness was something else. The boys, although chilly, thought that the weather was not all bad, as every school in the Highlands and Islands was closed.

When I had dressed and gathered courage, I went outside, carrying some hot water to melt the ice on the chickens' water bowl and to feed them. Although they had a well-insulated house, the two hens roosting near the door had succumbed to the cold. Needless to say, there were no eggs.

The weather was so unusual for Papavray that the whole

atmosphere seemed weird. The sky was a uniform grey: it had a brittle, crackly feel and the freezing mist of morning formed airborne ice particles that burned one's face. It was eerily quiet and nothing moved. No blast of the belligerent wind, no drumming of rain on the roofs, no bellowing of cattle or barking of dogs. Not a voice, not a car, not a tractor disturbed the uncanny silence. This was no crisp, frosty morning when one could take appreciative lungfuls of clear, cold air. A gulp of air today would burn lips, search out loose fillings and sear protesting lungs. The hills themselves seemed bowed with the weight of the freezing air, and everything appeared to be in a state of suspended animation, just waiting until the grinding, oppressing, all-pervading cold should lift.

But there was no snow, just ice and cold. Taps refused to run, wells froze solid and the burn was a tumble of ice and rocks. It broadened into a pool near our boundary and by using a crowbar and kettles of hot water we were able to lower buckets into the icy depths. By the time we had carried one back across the croft to the house and returned for another a thin layer of ice had already begun to form in the hole.

As I staggered indoors from the chicken house, Archie appeared, sliding and puffing his way across the croft.

'Mary-J!' he shouted, and his voice, normally blown away by the wind, sounded clear and crisp in the still air. 'My, my!' he exclaimed breathlessly. 'It's cold, cold indeed.' He seemed set for a chat, so I interrupted.

'Archie, it's far too cold to stand here. Come in, for goodness' sake!'

Thankfully, we stood close to the Rayburn. At the opposite end of the open-plan room, the boys were at the hearth with newspaper, sticks, coal and peat. They seemed to be building the 'towering inferno', and I began to think that we might get warm today after all.

Archie was speaking, '. . . and I'm off in the boat, y'see, so give me a list of any shopping you need. Not too much, mind! Only what you need. There'll be plenty will need things. You'll get milk and eggs anyway from Old Roderick, but he has nothin else left in his wee shop. Tis all gone!'

I began to understand that Archie was going round the coast to Dalhavaig by boat.

The icy roads over Ben Criel and by Loch Annan were impassable, the low clouds adding more and more frozen layers to the thick ice already covering their surfaces, so the only way out of the village for much-needed supplies was now by boat.

I dragged my mind back to Archie. 'I think you are very brave, Archie.'

Much embarrassed, he replied, 'Ach, tis nothin! Nothin at all. Sea's like a millpond. Your phone workin, is it?'

Surprised at the change of subject, I answered, 'Yes. Amazingly it is.'

'Ah,' he said.

'What is it, Archie? Something bothering you?'

'Well, two things. When I get to Dalhavaig, I'll be ringin you to send Nick across to tell Mary I'm safe.' (So, although Archie sounded confident, Mary was obviously not happy with this intended boat trip.) He continued, 'And I'm hearin that the wee girl is no well at Struakin.'

'Fiona! Oh my!' Struakin would be totally cut off at the moment. Sarah, Robbie and Fiona were the only folk there now, and they were about to move away.

'How do you know this, Archie?'

He began to look sheepish and shuffled his feet. I realised that he had been indulging in a hobby of his – listening in to the police and emergency radio bands on his old transistor. 'What is happening about it?'

'I'm thinkin Dr Mac might have got through on the phone, but I think there is something wrong with that too.'

After he had gone, with a short list of necessities (I had a huge, well-stocked freezer), I rang Dr Mac.

'I don't know, Nurse,' he said in answer to my questions. 'The line is so poor, but I keep trying to get through.' Thinking of my helicopter friends, I asked if they were an option if it was an emergency.

'They'll not get a helicopter even if it is urgent. There's freezing fog on the mainland and they can't take off. And there's no way I can drive to the end of the road, and, even supposing I could, I'm too old and too arthritic to walk that two-mile track. I'll just keep trying to get through.'

A moment or two later, the phone rang. It was John, our policeman.

'Nurse! Stop Archie from leaving NOW and then ring me!'

Taken aback but galvanised by such a peremptory tone, I grabbed a coat and raced outside. I could see a figure plodding towards the old boathouse where the local men kept their nets and outboard engines. Suddenly glad of the still conditions, I yelled his name and, in spite of the distance, he heard and turned back. Together we returned to the house, where I phoned John.

'Doctor finally spoke to Sarah. He wants you to go with Archie and ask him to put you ashore at Struakin, and once there you are to look after Fiona until the inshore lifeboat arrives from the mainland and then accompany them to the hospital. Doc thinks it's appendicitis. All right?'

'Yes, yes!' was all that I could think of to say. Archie had gathered what was needed. Regretfully, I looked at the huge fire, which was beginning to heat the house at last. I donned the warmest clothes to hand (bother the uniform) and followed Archie to the boathouse.

We pulled and pushed the heavy, clinker-built boat into the inky, undulating water, and he began to wrestle with the cold engine. After much muttering and energetic tugging at the starter cord, there was a cough, a splutter, a satisfying roar and we were off.

The trip was smooth and uneventful but unbelievably cold. Cutting through the sea at quite a speed, we were creating our own rushing wind, which made it even colder. I soon abandoned the seat and slid into the well of the boat. At least it was fractionally warmer there. How Archie managed to keep his head up and his blue, distance-focused eyes open and fixed ahead was a mystery to me, but he seemed completely at ease.

We rounded a headland and the little ruined harbour of Struakin came into sight. Robbie was on the shore to meet us as Archie cut the engine and we slid through the shallow water to ground gently on the pebbles.

Robbie was distraught. 'She is in so much pain, Mary-J. Down here.' He indicated an area on the lower right-hand side of his abdomen.

'When is the lifeboat likely to be here?' I asked.

'About an hour now, I should think.'

One hour! And then another perhaps to load and take Fiona to the hospital. I was worried, knowing how a patient's condition can change almost from minute to minute in some cases, and an appendix can burst without warning.

We followed Robbie into the house. The phone was ringing.

Sarah answered and passed it to me. The inshore lifeboat had left the mainland some half an hour ago and so should be here in another 20 to 30 minutes depending on the fog. Apparently it was getting worse, and I was told to have 'contingency plans' should they be late or, indeed, unable to get there at all.

'You do know that we are very isolated, with virtually no other way out of here and that we do not have the doctor's help?' I was really worried now.

'Of course! But we can't work miracles. There must be another boat there, surely?'

Archie! He was still hovering around. I would keep him and his precious boat here if I could.

I went into the bedroom. A hot, flushed face gazed at me from the snowy pillow. Fiona had been crying but was quiet at the moment while Sarah gently bathed her forehead.

'Hello, Fiona.'

A weak smile answered me. I explained that I was about to 'have a look at her tummy'. I barely touched her abdomen but I could feel the 'guarding' of the muscles and she flinched. Her temperature was up, as was her pulse rate.

'I think Dr Mac is probably right, Sarah.'

'Rob will have to go with her in the lifeboat. I get so seasick that I'd just be a nuisance, Mary-J.'

I was hoping that the fog would lift and that the lifeboat would be able to get here, as the thought of poor Fiona going in Archie's boat was not a happy one. It would be cold, uncomfortable and the jolting dangerous, but anything was better than doing nothing. Archie, however, was getting restless.

'Nurse. If I don't go soon, I'll not get back by dark.'

At that moment we heard the roar of powerful engines. Rob came running into the house.

'Off we go!' He was trying to be jolly and, wrapping the little girl in a warm blanket, lifted her gently and effortlessly and carried her out into the freezing weather. The inshore lifeboat was rocking quietly on the tide line. Fiona was made comfortable and strapped in. She lay among cushions, cocooned in blankets and waterproofs.

Archie had raised a hand in salute and was now speeding away through the water on his way to complete his interrupted shopping trip.

Robbie sat protecting Fiona from the wind and off we went. I felt that my presence was achieving nothing, for what could I do? He was a big, strong man to hold her and carry her and, although obviously in pain, she was quiet and comforted by his presence. But Archie had gone and my instructions had been to accompany the patient.

We were not travelling at full speed, as the crew recognised the need for a smooth ride, but the land swell rocked the boat alarmingly. We had to keep as close to the shore as the outcrops of rocks and small islets would allow because of the dense, patchy, swirling fog farther out to sea.

Very soon, we rounded the last headland and came within sight of Dalhavaig. The airborne bows sank to sea level as we slowed and slid into the harbour. The ambulance was waiting and Fiona was transferred to the elderly vehicle.

The road from the waterfront to the hospital had been scraped and sanded by the busy roadman, Charlie! As always, Joc was with his master. As the ambulance passed, Charlie stood to attention and saluted. I found this gesture of concern and respect very touching. He would have been told by the ambulance driver, or perhaps Archie, that it was Fiona who was ill and in all probability what the diagnosis was likely to be.

The vehicle lurched along and negotiated the slight rise to the hospital. I reported to the young surgeon, who wasted no time in taking Fiona through to the theatre.

With Fiona in good hands, I began to wonder how or even if I would get home. Perhaps Archie was still in the village? Perhaps I could get home with him? With a quick 'goodbye' to Rob, I set off towards the harbour.

A voice hailed me. 'Nurse! Tis you! You'll be looking for Archie.' It was Charlie. 'Aye, I ken you'd no be long up there. She'll be in the operation by now, I'm thinkin.'

'Yes, Charlie, she will be. Where is Archie? I'm hoping to catch a lift home with him.'

'Aye, I know. I told him he'd be as well to wait for ye. He's at the pier now. Look!'

And there he was in the distance, sitting in his boat, tied up to the pier.

I looked at Charlie in admiration. 'How did you know I'd be back and looking for a lift with him?' As soon as I had spoken, I thought how stupid I was to ask. It would be just another example of the efficiency of the jungle telegraph and the thoughtfulness of these island people.

'Ach,' said Charlie. 'Tis the sensible thing to do. But hurry! He'll not want to wait. The light will no be with us past three and tis gone midday.'

'Here she is then, Archie,' he announced on reaching the pier. It sounded as if he were delivering some long-awaited parcel. I scarcely had time to thank him before the engine spluttered into life and Archie turned the boat towards the mouth of the harbour.

'We'll be putting on a bit speed. We've not much time before dark.'

'Why are we going back this way? Surely the usual route is shorter than going back past Struakin again?'

Archie was embarrassed. 'Aye. Well, y'see, it was like this. While you were seein to the wee girl, Sarah asked me to get her a few wee things. What with her movin soon, she'd not much food in. It'll not take us long.'

'What a good fellow you are, Archie.' And I really meant it. What kindness I had encountered on this dreadful day.

'Aye, well . . .' Archie coughed.

So we beached once more at Struakin. The goods were delivered and off we went again. Dhubaig was as icily unwelcoming as ever as we pulled the boat up the beach in the deepening twilight. Looking forward to a fire and warm food, my mind turned again to poor Sarah, alone at Struakin on this dark, bitter night. I trudged wearily homeward in the gloom.

Luckily it turned out that Fiona's appendix had not ruptured in spite of all the tossing about that she (and it) had endured. She was home within a week and seemed happy and relaxed when I went to remove her stitches. Sarah was far more shattered than the little patient.

FORTY-ONE

Lucky Johnny Peg-Leg

The steely Hebridean winter had begun and so had the ceilidhs once more. So, in the savage wind of a Cimmerian night, our torches bobbed with others as we climbed up to Fergie's house. We could smell the acrid peat smoke that billowed from the chimney: welcoming and homely, but I knew that once full of people the room would become unbearably hot. It seemed to me that ceilidhs were not *ceilidhs* unless everyone was perspiring freely by the end of the evening.

Fergie 'H' sat toasting his toes in front of his peat fire with a smug, self-satisfied look on his face. Also seated at Fergie's fireside were Archie and Mary, Behag, Marion, Murdoch and other crofter friends.

'Well, Mary-J, and how is old Johnny today? I was after takin him some herring for his supper yesterday and he was gie poorly then, I'm thinkin.' Mary was anxious about the old man.

'I went to see him this morning and he seemed slightly better. He was having some of your herring for his dinner,' I replied.

Johnny was a wrinkled, one-legged man: the only person I had ever seen in the Western world with an old-fashioned wooden 'peg-leg'. He had been given countless opportunities to have a modern, state-of-the-art limb fitted but he stubbornly refused, whittling himself a new leg whenever his old one showed signs of wear. He was very tall, thin and loose-limbed: he looked as though he would come to pieces at any moment. At 89, and the oldest inhabitant on the island, he was now causing concern, being seriously ill for the first time that anyone could remember.

'He was coughin that bad yesterday that I thought he had the pulmoney,' declared Mary knowledgably.

No one corrected her. We were used to her unique vocabulary.

Archie appeared to be deep in thought as he helped himself to another dram of Fergie's whisky.

'O course, he's no rightly a Papavray man at all,' he averred.

We all looked at him in surprise, because a good half of Johnny's claim to local fame was that he was the oldest Papavrian on the island.

'No, indeed,' continued Archie, much gratified at our reaction. 'He was born on Rhuna and came here when he was a wee boy.'

'How are you knowin that?' Mary was intrigued. Here was something about a neighbour that she hadn't known!

Archie leaned forward. 'Twas Ally told Kirsty back in '53, when we was all in Donny and Marie's house for the weddin, y'mind.' He turned to us, 'Ally is Johnny's nephew. Big man, strong. Built like a horse.' As an afterthought, he added, 'He's dead now.'

'Aye,' said Fergie. 'I remember now. We were told that Johnny came over with his parents when they were "cleared" off Rhuna.'

'But that must have been in about . . .' I did some quick

calculation. 'It's '72 now, so it must have been 1880-something. I thought the Clearances were all over by then.'

Archie looked at me vaguely. 'Oh, maybe, maybe.' It was too good a story to be disproved by mere logic! Gaels preferred to stick to a good story, true or otherwise. If it were true, however, I realised that I actually knew someone who had been a subject of those infamous Clearances. Suddenly, past and present came together for me.

Fergie stirred. 'Aye, Johnny was lucky. Many of the folk on Rhuna had to emigrate.'

'Johnny was lucky again later, y'mind. Indeed, he was. Twas in the war,' said Archie.

'Which war?' asked Nick. At 14, he was becoming very interested in military history, a fascination that remains with him to this day.

'Bound to be the first,' said George. 'If you think about it, Nick, we're talking about an octogenarian.'

'Oh no,' piped Mary. 'Johnny was always Free Kirk.'

George was suddenly afflicted by a fit of coughing!

'Aye, twas the first, all right. Some place in France.'

'What happened?' George had recovered. And finally Archie began his tale.

'Well, he was out on patrol in some foreign part, lookin for Germans. "Mopping up" they called it, after the Germans had retreated. They found this gun emplacement and went inside, carefully enough, y'understand, to make sure all the Jerries had gone. They had begun to collect up food and ammunition and such, when there was an almighty explosion and they were all blown to glory! It was booby-trapped, y'see. Well, Johnny, he was blown up with all his mates. They were all killed. Johnny was wounded and near dead, too. Dear, dear, he was bad indeed. All night he was there, but in the morning the British came and found him and they got him to the field hospital. It seems his leg was that bad he got gangrene and they had to cut it off. The one he hasn't got, y'understand.' Archie liked to make things clear.

He continued, 'Apparently, they had run out of anaesthetic, so they had to do it without, because they didn't dare wait for new supplies. He would have died, y'see.' Archie paused, nodding. 'Aye, he was lucky, indeed.'

'Lucky' was not a word that I would readily have used to describe the fate of one suffering an amputation without anaesthetic!

'In the long term, it does not seem to have done him much harm in himself. After all, he has made 89 and he manages very well on his peg-leg,' I observed.

'I'd like to talk to him about the war and so on,' said Nick, much intrigued.

But he never did. Old Johnny went to meet his Maker that night.

At 3 a.m., the phone rang. It was Behag, Johnny's long-suffering daughter, herself in her late 60s, who had been looking after the irascible old man for many weeks now in his cottage by the harbour in Dalhavaig.

'Nurse! Tis Father. He's gone and died on me, just when I thought he was getting better.' She sounded aggrieved, but continued, 'He had even started to shout at me again. Last evening, I got him right for the night and then something made me go back in at midnight and there he was. Gone!'

'Behag, I'm so sorry. Have you told Dr Mac?'

'Aye, I have, but he says that it wasn't unexpected so he'll do the stificate on the morrow and that I was to ring you.'

'Where are you phoning from?' I knew that, in common with most of the crofters, she did not have a phone. Most of them professed to hate 'those contraptions'.

'From the post office in Dalhavaig.'

'Behag, why did you leave it for three hours before ringing me?'

'Well, Maggie gave me a wee cuppie and we got chattin . . .'

I couldn't believe my ears! They had sat chatting while Behag's father quietly slipped towards rigor mortis.

I dressed quickly, collected what I would need and departed into the night to fulfil my last obligation to Johnny.

*

The day of Johnny's funeral dawned cold, wet and windy, with menacing clouds racing across an angry sky. His burial service was to take place in his little croft house, and this was not unusual as that was where the 'corpus' would be lying. There was no such thing as a funeral parlour on Papavray, so funerals had to be arranged to take place within a few days of the death, as the croft houses were tiny and often occupied by a whole family. So distant relatives were telegraphed, the local women started baking and the men looked out fusty funeral suits.

Hailstones pattered on the windows of Johnny's little house during the service, while the howling gale and roaring sea accompanied the monotonous drone of the minister's voice. The squat house seemed to hunch its shoulders as gust after pugnacious gust raced in from the sea, whirled along the stone pier and thundered against the two-foot-thick walls. The wind found its way down the old chimney, covering the mourners in peaty smoke until our faces almost matched our sombre clothes. The Reverend McDuff coughed and spluttered his way through the devotions in the packed little room.

Johnny had been well known and a sizeable crowd had gathered, so that many of the men had to stand outside in the wind and the rain. As soon as the last 'amen' had been mumbled, the women started to brew gallons of tea and set out the clootie dumpling, cakes and oat biscuits, while the men, bearing the earthly remains of the old man, accompanied the minister to a little cemetery on the hill. In no time, they were back to crowd into the house once more, to eat and drink, chat and laugh whilst recalling Johnny's exploits. It was a very merry funeral indeed.

Suddenly, the door was flung open and a windswept figure bellowed at us, 'Can ye no hear the maroons? The coal boat's in bother! She's wallowin just outside the harbour.'

Everyone rushed for the door, jostling their way outside, and sure enough there was the familiar old tub flopping about on the turbulent waves. The wind was so strong that I had to hold on to the railings in order to stand up.

'She's lost her steerin,' asserted Fergie, fortissimo. 'She'll no get into the harbour. She's more likely to break up.'

I could see two crew members frantically clinging to the wheelhouse while the huge waves pounded against the harbour wall and bounced back to thunder over the deck. We could hear the crash of the hull as it was thrown against the wall time and time again.

'Where is her lifeboat?' I asked, with my mouth an inch or so from Fergie's ear. He looked at me as though I were mad.

'Ach, she has none. It would take up too much space. There'd be no room for the coal.'

On the pier, about 20 men set about throwing ropes to those

on the boat. We held our breath as one of the crew let go of the wheelhouse in order to grab one as the wind whipped it about over his head. He was knocked flat by a huge wave and was sliding towards the edge. The other man grabbed his legs and hauled him back to safety. He had nearly been washed over the side and would probably have been smashed to pieces between the hull and the harbour wall.

The rope was thrown again and this time the men on board the boat caught it and secured it round the capstan. All was now ready for the men on the quay to begin heaving and straining to try to steady the crazy pitching and rolling and turn the bows into the harbour entrance. A moment or two later, a shout went up as a higher than usual wave carried her into the gap. The heaving men tumbled over each other in the rush to reposition themselves and realign the ropes to bring her round and alongside.

About 30 minutes later, with tremendous effort and much shouting, she was being tied up in the comparative safety of the harbour. Many of the men were exhausted and sat on the wall, chests heaving. But even then their sense of humour surfaced and jokes about 'yon daft crew' were bandied about.

The 'daft crew' was amazingly unhurt and came ashore to partake of the remains of the funeral meal, which the women had brought to the wooden hut on the pier. I was busy for a long time in the confines of a dark, malodorous shack, treating blisters and cuts on the men's hands and arms. Being crofters and fishermen, they had rough, calloused skin already, but the ropes had been cold, wet and salty, and the amount of grip and pull that had been necessary to move the laden old craft had been phenomenal. There would be some sore muscles tomorrow!

After a while, I went back to Johnny's house and helped to

clear up. Everyone was talking of the day's adventures.

'Aye. We'll remember Johnny's funeral all right.'

'Indeed. And the coal boat. My, it's a good thing we was all here. If Johnny hadn't upped and died when he did, that boat would be at the bottom of the sea. And the crew with her, I wouldn't wonder. Aye. Twas lucky, foreby!'

So, even after he had 'passed over', Johnny was still spreading his luck.

FORTY-TWO

Fire!

Christmas was nearly upon us again! The need for one of our now-famous shopping expeditions became pressing, but at this time of the year it was virtually impossible to do it in one day as it was dark until about 10 a.m. and the light failed again by 3.30 p.m. So we were to stay with Angus and Maggie. Angus of the bottomless store! I wondered what monstrosity he might have for us to transport this time.

For several days before the intended trip, we watched the weather with anxiety. If it snowed heavily, Glen Knochiel would be impassable and our plans (and perhaps our Christmas) would be spoilt.

On the appointed day, armed with the usual enormously long shopping list (again as many things for others as for ourselves), we set off well before daylight. The weather was bitterly cold and snow was forecast. Mary was coming with us to stay with her cousins and have a 'good crack' (a gossip).

The shopping round followed the usual pattern, but with more time to spare it was much more enjoyable and we even visited the one and only theatre to see a performance of Dickens' *A Christmas Carol*. On the third day, as we prepared for our return, Mary announced that she had decided to stay for another few days.

'I'll come back with the Commission or the school inspector,' she said.

I was puzzled. She explained.

'I could get a lift with the school inspector, but I'm thinkin he's that clever he's no fun at all! No. I'll likely catch the Commission instead.'

'The Commission?' I repeated.

'Aye. He comes from the Crofters' Commission to inspect the land.'

'Do you know that he will take you?'

'Ach, he'll take me all right!' She nodded knowingly. 'Yon mannie will be after some venison from Archie.'

So all was clear! With grateful thanks to our hosts, and the Land Rover packed to the roof with everything from Christmas trimmings to a back boiler for hot water, we set off.

Mary had been scathing when she saw the back boiler. 'Can they no just boil a wee kettle full like other folk?'

I forbore to remind her that many folk, including ourselves, had baths and therefore needed rather more than a 'wee kettle full'!

Once away from the town, the snowy landscape opened up before us. The white hills, the dark green of the pine forests and the grey waters of the loch, ice-covered in places, were a perfect backdrop to the shaggy Highland cattle at the water's edge. Their thick coats were catching the huge snowflakes as they fell and when they raised their heads to inspect us they seemed to be wearing fluffy white hats.

The Highlands of Scotland are at their most spectacular in the snow. View after beautiful view opened up before us as we drove deeper and deeper into the wild landscape. Regal mountains, clothed in white, stood out against a leaden sky, but occasionally the clouds would part and silvery sunlight slanted across the shimmering slopes. The lonely scene glowed in the eerie light, while steely lochs reflected the sombre sky, the water appearing even darker at the edges where its gloom contrasted with the white banks. Vast pine forests shivered starkly under their white mantles, looking like so many thousands of Christmas trees. Craggy rocks beside the road were softened by the blanket of snow and young birch trees bowed their heads under the weight of the clinging flakes.

By the time we reached Papavray, the dim light of the winter day had dawdled imperceptibly into darkness and it was getting rapidly colder. I hoped we were not going to have a repeat of the intensely cold weather that we had experienced a few weeks ago.

With thoughts of home and a meal, and glad of the four-wheel-drive capability of the Land Rover, we climbed the dark, slippery side of Ben Criel.

'What's that smell?' asked Andy.

'It smells like a bonfire,' said Nick. 'There's red in the sky too. Look!'

We looked. An angry pink and red glow was spreading across the sky, interspersed with billowing black clouds. Clouds? No. This was smoke!

We came over the top of the hill, looking down on Loch Annan. George braked and we stared in amazement. We were among the high hills on the side of Ben Criel; hills that were now ablaze with roaring, crackling flames of orange and red shooting high into the air. They left a trail of sparks to be borne away on the fresh breeze and to alight on any nearby hill, possibly starting another fire.

We were speechless. There was an almost primeval magnificence about the awe-inspiring scene which left one feeling diminished, insignificant in the face of this exhibition of the power of nature's forces.

'It's the heather,' I said, in a sort of trance. 'It's so dry and brittle. We haven't had rain for weeks.'

The crofters lit controlled heather fires every three or four years, usually in February, normally a 'dry' month. If left undisturbed, the heather on the hills would become huge and woody, taking over the grazing intended for sheep and deer. With great skill, born of years of experience, 20 or so men with fire beaters would select an area of hillside – a different area each year – and set light to the heather in a long line, having determined the direction and strength of the wind. It was an organised and well-disciplined exercise.

But this was quite different. Magnificent to look at, maybe, but dangerous to the people fighting the fire and lethal to sheep caught in corries with flames all around them. And for much of the island's grazing to be destroyed could have serious economic effects.

For a few moments, we were mesmerised by the spectacle, viewed from our lofty perch, but speedily realised that we should be over there helping. Luckily, we always kept wellies in the vehicle, so we changed from our town shoes, pulling on extra sweaters, and were just setting off on foot when we were startled by the blast of a klaxon. The island's elderly fire engine lumbered past, travelling at a protesting 20 miles an hour. Long ago, the islanders had realised that they could not rely on a swift response to a 999 call and were apt to tackle any fire without recourse to the fire service at all. But this was a major conflagration that needed all the help available. The monstrous vehicle, which might once have been red, descended the hill with its brakes squealing and grinding. I could see six men packed into the cab.

As we followed on foot, I became aware of the rare sight of a shining, frozen Loch Annan surrounded by flames. The icy surface reflected the pink and grey clouds of smoke and the glowing hills, while the contrast between the silver loch and the brilliant colours of the roaring flames was spectacular.

The firemen were wrestling with hoses and pumps. Loch Annan would provide plenty of water now that the surface ice had been broken: some of the crofters had been wielding pickaxes. Then, to our utter amazement, we saw the factor's Land Rover crossing the loch towards the opposite hills – on the ice! I held my breath. How did Richard know that the ice was thick enough to take the weight of a Land Rover? Much later, when I asked him, he shrugged and said nonchalantly, 'I just hoped!' Crazy man! But he had a small generator and was trailing a hose to the inaccessible side of the loch so that a fireman, already in position, could direct the flow to the more remote areas of the fire.

As soon as we approached, we were given fire beaters – big floppy rubber flaps on stout poles – to whack the smouldering peaty ground. It had not really occurred to me that, just as peat burns in fireplaces so, after a dry, windy spell of weather, when the peaty ground is tinder dry, it would readily burn where it lay. The thought of the ground burning beneath your feet was horrific!

There was a modern house high in the hills near Loch Annan. No one knew how the absent owner had obtained planning permission to build out on common land but there it stood among the heather-clad, peaty soil. And now it was in grave danger. We, the family, were instructed to beat the hot, smouldering ground around 'yon daft house' and we were joined by many of the crofter women. Our feet became uncomfortable on the hot ground, and added to the smell of burning heather was a distinctly rubbery aroma. Our boots were beginning to melt!

About a dozen people saved 'yon daft house' from the fire that night while the sweating, exhausted men gradually subdued the flames on the hillsides. The firemen pumped water for hours to wherever they could reach, as did Richard until the generator broke down. Somewhere over the back of a hill a group of men lit a 'back fire' to provide a firebreak.

Gradually, the roaring and crackling subsided, the flames died to a pink glow and the fire was almost out. Men began to gather to consume vast quantities of tea, beer, water – anything that would quench their raging thirsts. They collapsed onto the ground, too tired to speak. Some of them had been there for six hours with no let-up in the filthy, back-breaking work. Many of the women, most of whom had been beating with us, dipped scarves into the loch where the ice had been smashed and attempted to wipe their smoke-grimed faces and hands.

It was midnight before it was decided that we should all go home. A number of men would be left behind to watch for any more outbreaks, due to the smouldering peat. The firemen rumbled off in a cloud of exhaust fumes and we started the long climb back to the Land Rover. We were black from head to toe and our boots had assumed an odd shape due to the heat. We were completely exhausted. We even had trouble climbing into the Land Rover and would still have to clean up before we could get to bed.

Surprisingly, after we had all showered and gathered by the Rayburn – we were too tired to light the fire – we felt refreshed.

After some hot soup, we all trailed upstairs to bed. But I was too tired to sleep and lay mulling over the night's events and thinking about the future. Would the weather allow Beth and Paul to come for Christmas? How were Nick and Andy progressing at school? Their reports were due soon. I hoped my new relief nurse would like the island and the work enough to stay: she was very young. Were John and Joanna really enjoying the Papavray life? And there was their baby to look forward to. I was to be a grandmother next spring!

I wondered what else the following years might hold for us all as I finally fell asleep on that cold winter night in our Hebridean home.

EPILOGUE

Just a dream?

I shall go back there one day. One day before I die.

I want to be there for the first winter gale, to hear the boom of the sea as it thunders among jagged rocks and beats against granite cliffs, as it surges into dark caverns, rattles over pebbles or rushes to meet chattering burns as they plunge to their salty destiny. I must watch again those foaming green waves crashing loudly and incessantly on the shore, while the wind whips spindrift high into the air and the tiny fishing boats toss wildly in the restless water.

I can almost see the snow on Ben Criel, the ice on Loch Annan and the tall plumes of peat smoke rising from little white croft houses in the still frosty air. I want to smell again the heather and bog myrtle, feel soft summer rain on my face and watch the fierce fire of a setting sun as it paints the sky with orange, gold and crimson light, lending its mirrored glory to the sea and its surreal splendour to the shimmering slopes of distant mountains. Later, I would be left in the peace of the long Northern twilight, to dream of the days when we lived and loved and worked in this blessed place.

Will I ever again sit in a cottage kitchen and share a 'cuppie' with a crofter's wife as I used to do? Or perhaps taste the oatmeal porridge that only Scots can cook to perfection? And talk once more with the dear, unique people who still live on that remote, rocky isle?

I wonder if I shall ever travel on the little steamer to the stone pier at Dalhavaig, or drive over high, undulating roads beside peat hags, or walk on the shore at Dhubaig, listening to stags roaring high in the hills. Shall I see the croft house in which we lived so long ago? Or hear skylarks heralding the spring or watch greylag geese as skein after skein comes home to Papavray? Perhaps it's just a dream.

Once we had a different dream and that one came true. We spent many wonderful years in this Hebridean sanctuary. How long ago was it? So much has happened since those far off days, but a lasting love of Papavray and the music of memory beckon me back. But perhaps that is all that I will ever have: memories of that Hebridean island. At least I have those, and they will do for now.

Glossary

Ben or Bheinn   a mountain

besom   an irritating, unpleasant woman

bodach   an old man

burn   a small stream often fast-flowing and stony

byre   a stone barn

cailleach   an old woman (often wife), not necessarily derogatory

ceilidh   (1) a neighbourly gathering in each other's houses for food, drink and entertainment (amateur but often very accomplished) (2) a large, organised dance arranged for the tourists

Ciamar a tha   Hello, how are you?

clootie dumpling   a pudding made in a cloth (the cloot) and boiled. It contains flour, suet, dried fruit, oats and sugar

lum   chimney

loch   a lake – may be freshwater inland or sea loch

peat   decomposed vegetable matter, laid down thousands of years ago, mainly in the acidic soil of Scotland, Ireland and other countries, dug for fuel (or gardens)

peat hag   an area of peat bog which has been delineated for rental

sheiling   rough shelter for crofters on the high summer grazing.

strupak   tea and a bite (and a gossip)

Tha gu math   Fine, thanks. How are you?